MENTAL HEALTH–SUBSTANCE USE

Developing Services in Mental Health–Substance Use

Edited by

DAVID B COOPER

Sigma Theta Tau International: The Honor Society of Nursing Award
Outstanding Contribution to Nursing Award
Editor-in-Chief, Mental Health and Substance Use: dual diagnosis
Author/Writer/Editor

Radcliffe Publishing
Oxford • New York

Radcliffe Publishing Ltd
18 Marcham Road
Abingdon
Oxon OX14 1AA
United Kingdom

www.radcliffepublishing.com
Electronic catalogue and worldwide online ordering facility.

British Library Cataloguing in Publication Data

A catalogue record for this book is available from the British Library.

ISBN-13: 978 184619 340 8

The paper used for the text pages of this book is FSC certified. FSC (The Forest Stewardship Council) is an international network to promote responsible management of the world's forests.

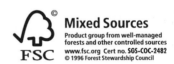

Mixed Sources
Product group from well-managed forests and other controlled sources
www.fsc.org Cert no. SGS-COC-2482
© 1996 Forest Stewardship Council

Typeset by Pindar NZ, Auckland, New Zealand
Printed and bound by TJI Digital, Padstow, Cornwall, UK

Developing Services in Mental Health–Substance Use

Contents

Preface

Approximately six years ago Phil Cooper, then an MSc student, was searching for information on mental health–substance use. At that time, there was one journal and few published papers. This led to the launch of the journal *Mental Health and Substance Use: dual diagnosis*, published by Taylor and Francis International. To launch the journal, and debate the concerns and dilemmas of psychological, physical, social, legal and spiritual professionals, Phil organised a conference for Suffolk Mental Health NHS Trust and Taylor and Francis. The response was excellent. An occurring theme was that more information, knowledge and skills were needed – driven by education and training.

Discussion with international professionals indicated a need for this type of educational information and guidance, in this format, and a proposal was submitted for one book. The single book progressed to become a series of six! The concept is that each book will follow on from the other to build a sound basis – as far as is possible – of the important approaches to mental health–substance use. The aim is to provide a 'how to' series that will be interactive with case studies, reflective study and exercises – you, as individuals and professionals, will decide if this has been achieved.

So, why do we need to know about mental health–substance use? International concerns related to interventions, and the treatment of people experiencing mental health–substance use problems, are frequently reported. These include:
- 'the most challenging clinical problem that we face'[1]
- 'substance misuse is usual rather than exceptional amongst people with severe mental health problems'[2]
- 'Mental health and substance use problems affect every local community throughout America'[3]
- 'The existence of psychiatric comorbidities in young people who abuse alcohol is common, especially for conditions such as depression, anxiety, bipolar disorder, conduct disorder and attention-deficit/hyperactivity disorder'[4]
- 'Mental and neurological disorders such as depression, schizophrenia, epilepsy and substance abuse . . . cause immense suffering for those affected, amplify people's vulnerability and can lead individuals into a life of poverty'.[5]

There is a need to appreciate that mental health–substance use is now a concern for us all. This series of books will bring together what is known (to some), and what is not (to some). If undertaken correctly, and you, the reader will be the judge – and those individuals you come into contact with daily will be the final judges – each book will build on the other and be of interest for the new, and the not so new, professional.

The desire to provide services that facilitate best practice for mental health–substance use is not new. The political impetus for this approach to succeed now exists. We, the professionals, need to seize on this momentum. We need to bring about the much-needed change for the individual who experiences our interventions and treatment, be that political will because of a perceived financial benefit or, as we would hope, the need to provide therapeutic interventions for the individual. Whatever the motive, now is the time to grasp the initiative.

Before we (the professionals) can practice, research, educate, manage, develop or purchase services, we must commence with knowledge. From that, we begin to understand. We commence using our new-found skills. We progress to developing the ability to examine practice, to put concepts together, to make valid judgements. We achieve this level of expertise though education, training and experience. Sometimes, we can use our own life experiences to enhance our skills. But knowledge must come first, though is often relegated to last! Professionals (from health, social, spiritual and legal backgrounds) – be they students, practitioners, researchers, educators, managers, service developers or purchasers – are all 'professionals' (in the eye of the individual we meet professionally), though each has differing depths of knowledge, skills and expertise.

What we need to remember is that the individual (those we offer care to), family and carers bring their own knowledge, skills and life experiences – some developed from dealing with ill health. The individual experiences the illness, lives with it, manages it – daily. Therefore, to bring the two together, individual and professional, to make interventions and treatment outcome effective, to meet whatever the individual feels is acceptable to his or her needs, requires mutual understanding and respect. The professionals' skills and expertise '*are founded on nothing less than their complete and perfect acceptance of one, by another*'.[6]

David B Cooper
August 2010

REFERENCES

1 Appleby L. *The National Service Framework for Mental Health: five years on*. London: Department of Health; 2004. Available at: www.dh.gov.uk/prod_consum_dh/groups/dh_digitalassets/@dh/@en/documents/digitalasset/dh_4099122.pdf (accessed 25 February 2010).

2 Department of Health. *Mental Health Policy Implementation Guide: dual diagnosis good practice guide*. 2002. Available at: www.substancemisuserct.co.uk/staff/documents/dh_4060435.pdf (accessed 25 February 2010).

3 Substance Abuse and Mental Health Service Administration. *Results from the 2008 National Survey on Drug Use and Health*. 2008. Available at: www.oas.samhsa.gov/nsduh/2k8nsduh/2k8Results.cfm (accessed 25 February 2010).

4 Australian Government. *Australian Guidelines to Reduce Health Risks from Drinking Alcohol*.

2009. Available at: www.nhmrc.gov.au/publications/synopses/ds10syn.htm (accessed 25 February 2010).

5 World Health Organization. *Mental Health Improvements for Nations Development: the WHO MIND Project.* 2008. Available at: www.who.int/mental_health/policy/en (accessed 25 February 2010).

6 Thompson F. *Lark Rise to Candleford: a trilogy.* London: Penguin Modern Classics; 2009.

About the Mental Health–Substance Use series

The six books in this series are:
1 *Introduction to Mental Health–Substance Use*
2 *Developing Services in Mental Health–Substance Use*
3 *Responding in Mental Health–Substance Use*
4 *Intervention in Mental Health–Substance Use*
5 *Care in Mental Health–Substance Use*
6 *Practice in Mental Health–Substance Use*

The series is not merely for mental health professionals but also the substance use professionals. It is not a question of 'them' (the substance use professional) teaching 'them' (the mental health professional). It is about sharing knowledge, skills and expertise. We are equal. We learn from each fellow professional, for the benefit of those whose lives we touch. The rationale is that to maintain clinical excellence, we need to be aware of the developments and practices within mental health and substance use. Then, we make informed choices; we take best practice, and apply this to our professional role.[1]

Generically, the series *Mental Health–Substance Use* concentrates on concerns, dilemmas and concepts specifically interrelated, as a collation of problems that directly or indirectly influence the life and well-being of the individual, family and carers. Such concerns relate not only to the individual but also to the future direction of practice, education, research, service development, interventions and treatment. While presenting a balanced view of what is best practice today, the books aim to challenge concepts and stimulate debate, exploring all aspects of the development in treatment, intervention and care responses, and the adoption of research-led best practice. To achieve this, they draw from a variety of perspectives, facilitating consideration of how professionals meet the challenges now and in the future. To accomplish this we have assembled leading, international professionals to provide insight into current thinking and developments, from a variety of perspectives, related to the many varying and diverse needs of the individual, family and carers experiencing mental health–substance use.

REFERENCE

1 Cooper DB. Editorial: decisions. *Ment Health Subst Use.* 2010; **3**: 1–3.

About the editor

David B Cooper
Sigma Theta Tau International: Honor Society of Nursing Award
Outstanding Contribution to Nursing Award
Editor-in-Chief: *Mental Health and Substance Use: dual diagnosis*
Author/Writer/Editor

The editor welcomes approaches and feedback, positive and/or negative.

David has specialised in mental health and substance use for over 30 years. He has worked as a practitioner, manager, researcher, author, lecturer and consultant. He has served as editor, or editor-in-chief, of several journals, and is currently editor-in-chief of *Mental Health and Substance Use: dual diagnosis*. He has published widely and is '*credited with enhancing the understanding and development of community detoxification for people experiencing alcohol withdrawal*' (Nursing Council on Alcohol; Sigma Theta Tau International citations). Seminal work includes *Alcohol Home Detoxification and Assessment* and *Alcohol Use*, both published by Radcliffe Publishing, Oxford.

List of contributors

CHAPTER 2 **Dr Kevin Morgan**
Specialist Registrar in Addictions
Community Drug and Alcohol Service
London, UK

Kevin completed basic training in psychiatry at the Maudsley Hospital, London, following which he has worked in a number of substance-misuse and general psychiatry services within London. He has an interest in substance misuse disorders in the elderly and the psychiatry of old age in general. Other interests are the historical and social aspects of psychiatry and fiction writing.

Dr Karim Dar
Consultant Psychiatrist in Addictions
Gatehouse Alcohol Clinic
St Bernards Hospital
Southall, Middlesex, UK

Karim is Consultant Psychiatrist and Lead Clinician at the CNWL NHS Foundation Trust, London. He has responsibility for an inpatient detoxification unit (Max Glatt Unit) and a community alcohol team. He is especially interested in substance misuse problems in special populations and service development. He was an award holder in the Health Foundation UK national Leaders for Change programme and has a postgraduate qualification in health economics from the University of York.

CHAPTER 3 **Dr Alexander Baldacchino**
Clinical Senior Lecturer in Addiction Psychiatry, University of Dundee
Consultant Psychiatrist in Addictions, National Health Service Fife
Centre for Addiction Research and Education Scotland (CARES), Centre for Neuroscience, Division of Pathology and Neurosciences
Ninewells Hospital and Medical School
Dundee, UK

Alex has been researching comorbid substance misuse and associated psychiatric and physical issues for the last 15 years. His studies involved biological, neuropsychological, clinical, and policy-related research. In the last 10 years, he has been the UK Principal Investigator to several European Union funded projects. These include looking at barriers and challenges faced by individuals with substance misuse-related problems accessing treatment (IATPAD Study), a cross-cultural multicentre study to determine the nature, extent and management of drug-related mental health problems in Europe (Drugs and Psychosis and ISADORA Studies), Internet and drug addiction (Psychonaut 2002 study) among others. He is Director for the Centre of Addiction Research and Education Scotland (CARES), which is based at Ninewells Hospital Medical School.

Professor Ilana B Crome
Academic Clinical Director in Psychiatry
Consultant Psychiatrist in Addiction
Academic Psychiatry Unit
Keele University Medical School
South Staffordshire and Shropshire Healthcare NHS Foundation Trust
Stafford, UK

Ilana is one of only three professors of Addiction Psychiatry in the United Kingdom. Her clinical base is at South Staffordshire and Shropshire Foundation Trust, St George's Hospital, Stafford. Her interest and expertise in the field of comorbidity has informed the Department of Health and ACMD across the treatment, research and policy domains and this has been acknowledged by appointment to the NICE Guideline Development Group on Mental Illness and Substance Misuse. She is past President of the Alcohol and Drugs Section of the European Psychiatric Association, International Editor of *American Journal on Addictions* and Joint Editor of *Drugs: Education, Prevention and Policy.*

CHAPTER 4   Tom C Dodd
Joint National Programme Lead for Dual Diagnosis
National Primary Care Lead
National Institute for Mental Health in England
Northants, UK

Tom has led a number of national programmes including Community Teams, Primary Care and Dual Diagnosis. He currently divides his time as Commissioning and Developments Lead for 'Improving Access to Psychological Therapies' and Dual Diagnosis. Previously, he was with the Sainsbury Centre for Mental Health, where he helped to develop and lead work around Assertive Outreach Teams and crisis teams, with a focus on more severe and lasting mental health problems. He is a mental health nurse who has worked as a senior manager and led and established clinical teams in the NHS. He is passionate about carers' issues, and about how services work with families. For five years he was the chair of a charity, which he founded, that worked to improve well-being and reduce suicide in rural communities.

Ann Gorry
Joint National Programme Lead for Dual Diagnosis

National Institute for Mental Health in England
Northants, UK

Ann is a mental health nurse and has worked in alcohol/substance use services for most of her long and varied career. She set up a specialist dual diagnosis service in Cheshire 10 years ago and since then has worked in a number of senior clinical and managerial positions. In recent years, Ann has worked as a regional dual diagnosis lead, and for the past five years in a national role, and currently works as national dual diagnosis lead with the National Mental Health Development Unit. Ann is passionate about improving services for people who experience difficulties with alcohol/substance use and mental health, their carers and families. Much of her regional and national work has involved service users and carers with a particular focus on involvement in training and improving the confidence and capabilities of the workforce.

CHAPTER 5   **Dr Hermine L Graham**
Consultant Clinical Psychologist and Lecturer
School of Psychology
University of Birmingham
Birmingham and Solihull Mental Health NHS Foundation Trust
Birmingham, UK

Hermine previously developed and evaluated an integrated treatment approach for people with severe mental health problems who use substances problematically, as Head of the COMPASS Programme in Birmingham, prior to her current post. She has published within this area and provides consultancy on service and policy developments. Her research interests include the relationship between problematic substance use and psychosis, the application of cognitive therapy to this client group and cannabis use among young people. Hermine co-edited the book *Substance Misuse in Psychosis* (2003), and wrote the treatment manual *Cognitive-behavioural Integrated Treatment* (2004).

CHAPTER 6   **Gary J Croton**
Clinical Nurse Specialist
Northeast Health Wangaratta
Eastern Hume Dual Diagnosis Service
Victoria, Australia

Gary, a psychiatric nurse, has worked in mental health and drug treatment settings in Australia and the UK for 35 years. Since 1998 he has worked in a dedicated mental health–substance use capacity building role as the sole worker for Eastern Hume Dual Diagnosis Service (EHDDS) in rural NE Victoria, Australia. Gary has authored a range of manuals, fellowship reports, submissions, articles and book chapters around mental health–substance use and is the creator and webmaster of www.dualdiagnosis.org.au.

CHAPTER 7   Dr Diana PK Roeg
Senior Researcher
Tilburg University
Department of Tranzo
LE Tilburg, the Netherlands

Diana studied health sciences and specialised on health services research. She works as a postdoctoral researcher at Tilburg University, the Netherlands, in the department of Tranzo, the University's scientific centre for the transformation of the nature and quality of care and welfare. Tranzo universities and healthcare institutions collaborate to carry out long-term research programmes and to develop a knowledge infrastructure. Diana's dissertation was on the history and development of intensive community-based care. She developed an instrument to characterise programs in this sector. Recent research is into the effectiveness of intensive community-based care.

Dr Theo JM Kuunders
Health Policy Professional, Regional Public Health Service Centre
Science Practitioner/PhD Student
Public Health at Tranzo, Tilburg University
GGD Hart voor Brabant
VLs-Hertogenbosch, the Netherlands

Theo worked as a social psychiatric care provider for several mental health organisations. He studied Philosophy and ethics of care at the Radboud University Nijmegen, the Netherlands. His current profession is at the Municipal Public Health Centre, GGD Hart voor Brabant, where he advises local health policy for municipal authorities. Here he is also involved in coaching teams in outreaching interferential care. As a science practitioner he works at Tranzo, Tilburg University, bridging the gap between public health and scientific institutions.

CHAPTER 8   Dr Elizabeth Hughes
Reader in Mental Health/Substance Use Research
Faculty of Health and Life Science
Coventry University, Coventry, UK
Honorary Senior Research Fellow
Health Service and Population Research Department
Institute of Psychiatry, King's College London, UK

Liz has a background mental health nursing and has worked clinically in both substance use and mental health settings. She developed a dual diagnosis service in South East London, before taking up an academic post at the Institute of Psychiatry, King's College, London. Here she was involved in research and teaching related to dual diagnosis and psychosocial interventions for psychosis. In addition, she managed a London-wide dissemination project for dual diagnosis training to mental health workers across all London Trusts. In 2006, Liz moved to the University of

Lincoln where she undertook a pilot study of dual diagnosis training in prisons, the development of national framework for dual diagnosis capabilities, the development of an advanced module of the 10 Essential Shared Capabilities for dual diagnosis, and a team training resource for dual diagnosis aimed at Assertive Outreach Teams. Liz has presented and published widely in the area of mental health, dual diagnosis and health behaviour. Current projects include the development and evaluation of a national e-learning resource for dual diagnosis awareness.

CHAPTER 9   Amanda J Barrett
Service Manager: Dual Diagnosis
Tees, Esk and Wear Valleys NHS Foundation Trust
Middlesbrough, UK

Mandy qualified as an RMN in 1989 and has specialised in dual diagnosis since 2004, leading the County Durham Dual Diagnosis Project, featured in the Turning Point Dual Diagnosis Good Practice Handbook. Her qualifications include a BSc in Managing Health Care Delivery, a MA in Drug Interventions, and non-medical prescribing. Mandy's published work includes an article in *Journal of Substance Misuse*, a chapter in the book *Drugs in Britain* and an article in *Nursing Times*. Mandy was a member of the National CSIP Steering Group, which developed the dual diagnosis capabilities framework.

CHAPTER 10   Philip A Cooper
Nurse Consultant: Dual Diagnosis
5 Boroughs Partnership NHS Foundation Trust
Whiston, Merseyside, UK

Phil has worked in both substance misuse and mental health services over the last 15 years. He has developed training programmes regarding mental health–substance use and has been instrumental in developing proactive measures to address substance misuse in acute mental health settings in the North West of England. Phil has been active in supporting the development of a drop-in group for people with mental health–substance use issues and developing a format to assess intoxication levels when people present to mental health services.

CHAPTER 11   Professor Stephen R Onyett
Director, Steve Onyett Consultancy Services
Senior Development Consultant, South West Development Centre
Visiting Professor, University of the West of England
Bristol, UK

Steve's work on leadership and team development and coaching has taken him from heading clinical psychology services into a variety of roles in both provider and commissioning organisations. He specialises in solution-focused approaches to development that build sustainable and enjoyable relationships and work from the best that people bring to any situation. Steve currently leads on leadership and teamwork development for the South West Development Centre and runs his own successful consultancy (www.steveonyett.co.uk) offering solution-focused coaching, facilitation, research and training. Most of his work to date has been in health and social care, and he is an associate of Bristol Business School, visiting professor at the Faculty of Health and Life Sciences, University of the West of England and co-editor of the *International Journal of Leadership in Public Services*. He has published widely, including books on successful books on teamwork. Recent projects have included founding a leadership programme for social care leaders in the South West, a national survey of Home Treatment Teams and the Developing Effective Local Leadership for Social Inclusion initiative as part of the National Social Inclusion Programme.

CHAPTER 13   Professor Christopher CH Cook

Professorial Research Fellow; Tutor in Pastoral Studies
Cranmer Hall, St John's College, Durham
Consultant in Substance Use
Tees, Esk and Wear Valley NHS Foundation Trust
Durham, UK

Chris trained at St George's Hospital Medical School, London, and has worked in the psychiatry of substance misuse for 25 years. He was ordained as an Anglican priest in 2001. He is Director of the Project for Spirituality, Theology and Health at Durham University and an editor (with Andrew Powell and Andrew Sims) of *Spirituality and Psychiatry* (Royal College of Psychiatrists Press; 2009).

CHAPTER 14   Lyn Matthews

Drug and Alcohol Worker
The Armistead Centre
Liverpool, UK

Lyn has worked in the drugs field for 23 years and has worked for the Armistead Centre for the past six years. Throughout this time Lyn has specialised in issues around diversity. Lyn has contributed chapters and articles to both national and international publications. Lyn was part of the original team that developed the Mersey Model of Harm Reduction in the mid 80s, and developed and worked on one of the first outreach projects in Britain with street sex workers.

Jon Hibberd

Hospice Community Nurse Specialist
St Peter's Hospice
North Team
Bristol, UK

Jon qualified as a registered nurse in 1996. After a period of working as a Community Staff Nurse he went on to study for a BSc (Hons) degree in Community Healthcare Nursing. Jon then moved to North Devon where initially he worked as a Senior Staff

Nurse with the District Nursing Service. Jon then moved on to work at North Devon Hospice. For the first 18 months Jon undertook a Palliative Care Development Programme working both in the community as a Nurse Specialist, and in the day hospice. It was during this time Jon studied for the Diploma in Care of the Dying Patient. After this period Jon gained a full-time Community Nurse Specialist Post in Palliative Care position working in a large rural area within primary care. Recently, Jon moved to work at St Peter's Hospice, Bristol, as a Community Nurse Specialist.

CHAPTER 15 Dr Nicola Glover-Thomas
Reader in Law
The School of Law and Social Justice
University of Liverpool
Liverpool, UK

Nicola is a specialist in mental health law and more general medical law areas, particularly, pharmacy and pharmaceutical law. She has been engaged in research in these areas for the last 12 years and over more recent years has largely focused upon a socio-legal approach, often incorporating new empirical data. Her past work includes studies on the response of charities in housing the mentally vulnerable, and the use of off-label drugs in the care of children and young people with mental disorder. Currently, she is engaged in an empirical research project which examines the role of risk in mental health decision-making.

USEFUL CONTACTS Jo Cooper
Jo spent 16 years in specialist palliative care, initially working in a hospice in-patient unit, then 12 years as a Macmillan Clinical Nurse Specialist. She gained a Diploma in Oncology at Addenbrooke's Hospital, Cambridge, and a BSc (Hons) in Palliative Nursing at The Royal Marsden, London, and an Award in Specialist Practice. Jo edited *Stepping into Palliative Care* (2000) and the second edition, *Stepping into Palliative Care,* volumes 1 and 2 (2006), both published by Radcliffe Publishing. Jo has been involved in teaching for many years and her specialist subjects include management of complex pain and symptoms, terminal agitation, communication at the end of life, therapeutic relationships and breaking bad news.

Terminology

Whenever possible, the following terminology has been applied. However, in certain instances, when referencing a study and/or specific work(s), when an author has made a specific request, or for the purpose of additional clarity, it has been necessary to deviate from this applied 'norm.'

MENTAL HEALTH–SUBSTANCE USE

Considerable thought has gone in to the use of terminology within these texts. Each country appears to have its own terms for the person experiencing mental health and substance use problems – terms that includes words such as dual diagnosis, coexisting; co-occurring, and so on. We talk about the same thing but use differing professional jargon. The decision was set at the outset to use one term that encompasses mental health *and* substance use problems: *mental health–substance use*. One scholar suggested that such a term implies that both can exist separately, while they can also be linked.[1]

SUBSTANCE USE

Another challenge was how to term 'substance use'. There are a number of ways: abuse, misuse, dependence, addiction. The decision is that within these texts we use the term *substance use* to encompass all (unless specific need for clarity at a given point). It is imperative the professional recognises that while we may see another person's 'substance use' as misuse or abuse, the individual experiencing it may not deem it to be anything other than 'use'. Throughout, we need to be aware that we are working alongside unique individuals. Therefore, we should be able to meet the individual where he/she is.

ALCOHOL, PRESCRIBED DRUGS, ILLICIT DRUGS, TOBACCO OR SUBSTANCES

Throughout this book *substance* includes alcohol, prescribed drugs, illicit drugs and tobacco, unless specific need for clarity at a given point.

PROBLEM(S), CONCERNS AND DILEMMAS OR DISORDERS

The terms *problem(s)*, *concerns and dilemmas* and *disorders* can be used interchangeably, as stated by the author's preference. However, where possible, the term 'problem(s)' or 'concerns and dilemmas' had been adopted as the preferred choice.

INDIVIDUAL, PERSON, PEOPLE

There seems to be a need to label the individual – as a form of recognition! Sometimes the label becomes more than the person! 'Alan is schizophrenic' – thus it is Alan, rather than an illness that Alan lives with. We refer to patients, clients, service users, customers, consumers, and so on. Yet, we feel affronted when we are addressed as anything other than what we are – individuals! We need to be mindful that every person we see during our professional day is an individual – unique. Symptoms are in many ways similar (e.g. delusions, hallucinations), some need interventions and treatments are similar (e.g. specific drugs, psychotherapy techniques), but people are not. Alan may experience an illness labelled schizophrenia, and so may John, Beth and Mary, and you or I. However, each will have his/her own unique experiences – and life. None will be the same. To keep this constantly in the mind of the reader, throughout the book series we shall refer to the *individual, person* or *people* – just like us, but different to us by their uniqueness.

PROFESSIONAL

We are all professionals, whether students, nurses, doctors, social workers, researchers, clinicians, educationalists, managers, service developers, religious ministers – and so on. However, the level of expertise may vary from one professional to another. We are also individuals. There is a need to distinguish between the person with a mental health–substance use problem and the person interacting professionally (at whatever level) with that individual. To acknowledge and to differentiate between those who experience – in this context – and those who intervene, we have adopted the term *professional*. It is indicative that we have had, or are receiving, education and training related specifically to help us (the professionals) meet the needs of the individual. We may or may not have experienced mental health–substance use problems but we have some knowledge that may help the individual – an expertise to be shared. We have a specific knowledge that, hopefully, we wish to use to offer effective intervention and treatment to another human being. It is the need to make a clear differential, for the reader, that forces the use of 'professional' over 'individual' to describe our role – our input into another person's life.

REFERENCE

1 Barker P. Personal communication; 2009.

Cautionary note

Wisdom and compassion should become the dominating influence that guide our thoughts, our words, and our actions.[1]

Never presume that what you say is understood. It is essential to check understanding, and what is expected of the individual and/or family, with each person. Each person needs to know what he/she can expect from you, and other professionals involved in his/her care, at each meeting. Jargon is a professional language that excludes the individual and family. Never use it in conversation with the individual, unless requested to do so; it is easily misunderstood.

Remember, we all, as individuals, deal with life differently. It does not matter how many years we have spent studying human behaviour, listening and treating the individual and family. We may have spent many hours exploring with the individual his/her anxieties, fears, doubts, concerns and dilemmas, and the illness experience. Yet, we do not know what that person really feels, how he/she sees life and ill health. We may have lived similar lives, experienced the same illness but the individual will always be unique, each different from us, each independent of our thoughts, feelings, words, deeds and symptoms, each with an individual experience.

REFERENCE

1 Matthieu Ricard. As cited in: Föllmi D, Föllmi O. *Buddhist Offerings 365 Days*. London: Thames and Hudson; 2003.

Acknowledgements

I am grateful to all the contributors for having the faith in me to produce a valued text and I thank them for their support and encouragement. I hope that faith proves correct. Thank you to those who have commented along the way, and whose patience has been outstanding. Thank you to Jo Cooper, who has been actively involved with this project throughout – supporting, encouraging, listening and participating in many practical ways. Jo is my rock who looks after me during my physical health problems, and I am eternally grateful.

Many people have helped me along my career path and life – too many to name individually. Most do not even know what impact they have had on me. Some, however, require specific mention. These include Larry Purnell, a friend and confidant who has taught me never to presume – while we are all individuals with individual needs, we deserve equality in all that we meet in life. Thanks to Martin Plant (who sadly died in March 2010), and Moira Plant, who always encouraged and offered genuine support. Phil and Poppy Barker, who have taught me that it is OK to express how I feel about humanity – about people, and that there is another way through the entrenched systems in health and social care. Keith Yoxhall, without whose guidance back in the 1980s I would never have survived my 'Colchester work experience' and the dark times of institutionalisation, or had the privilege to work alongside the few professionals fighting against the 'big door'. He taught me that there was a need for education and training, and that this should be ongoing – also that the person in hospital or community experiencing our care sees us as 'professional' – we should make sure we act that way. Thank you to Phil Cooper, who brought the concept of this book series to me via a conference to launch the journal *Mental Health and Substance Use: dual diagnosis*, of which he was editor. It was then I realised that despite all the talk over too many years of my professional life, there was still much to be done for people experiencing mental health–substance use problems. Phil is a good debater, friend and reliable resource for me – thank you.

To Gillian Nineham of Radcliffe Publishing, my sincere thanks. Gillian had faith in this project from the outset and in my ability to deliver. Her patience is immeasurable and, for that, I am grateful. Thank you to Michael Hawkes for putting up with my too numerous questions! Thank you to Jamie Etherington, Editorial Development Manager, and Dan Allen of the book marketing department, both competent people who make my work look good. Thanks also to Mia Yardley and the production team at Pindar, New Zealand, for bringing this book to publication, and the many others who are nameless to me as I write but without whom these books would never come to print; each has his/her stamp on any successes of this book.

My sincere thanks to all of you named, and unnamed, my friends and colleagues along my sometimes broken career path: those who have touched my life in a positive way – and a few, a negative way (for we can learn from the negative to ensure we do better for others).

A final heartfelt statement: any errors, omissions, inaccuracies or deficiencies within these pages are my sole responsibility.

Dedication

This book is dedicated to Phil and Sarah. Phil is one of a special group of professionals who embraces the drive to improve the quality of care offered to the person experiencing mental health–substance use problems. Sarah, his partner, and fellow nurse, is Phil's soul mate. Phil is also my son of whom I am justifiably very proud!

CHAPTER 1

Setting the scene

David B Cooper

> *When it is obvious that the goals cannot be reached, don't adjust the goals, adjust the action steps.*[1]

PRE-READING EXERCISE 1.1

Time: 20 minutes

When preparing to read this book you may wish to undertake the following exercise.

Write a brief description of your thoughts and feelings in relation to mental health–substance use problems. When you have read the book repeat the exercise, taking note of the following:

- Have your thoughts and feelings changed? If yes, in what way?
- What information do you feel most influenced that change? What did not?
- Are there any areas that you feel you need to investigate further? If yes, what are they? What resources will you need?
- Make a plan of action to develop your learning and understanding of mental health–substance use.

INTRODUCTION

The difficulties encountered by people who experience mental health–substance use problems are not new. The individual using substances presenting to the mental health professional can often encounter annoyance and suspicion. Likewise, the person experiencing mental health problems presenting to the substance use services can encounter hostility and hopelessness. 'We cannot do anything for the substance use problem until the mental health problem is dealt with!' The referral to the mental health team is returned: 'We cannot do anything for this person until the substance use problem is dealt with!' Thus, the individual is in the middle of two professional worlds and neither is willing to move, and yet, both professional worlds are involved in 'caring' for the individual.

For many years, it has been acknowledged that the two parts of the caring system need to work as one. However, this desire has not developed into practice.

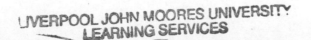

Over recent years, this impetus has changed. There is now a drive towards meeting the needs of the individual experiencing mental health–substance use problems, pooling expertise from both sides. Moreover, there is an international political will to bring about change, often driven forward by a small group of dedicated professionals at practice level.

Some healthcare environments have merely paid lip service, ensuring the correct terminology is included within the policy and procedure documentation, while at the same time doing nothing, or little, to bring about the changes needed at the practice level to meet the needs of the individual. Others have grasped the drive forward and have spearheaded developments at local and national level within their country to meet such needs. It appears that the latter are now succeeding. There is a concerted international effort to improve the services provided for the individual, and a determination to pool knowledge and expertise. In addition, there is the ability of these professional groups to link into government policy and bring about the political will to support such change. However, this cannot happen overnight. There are major attitudinal changes needed – not least at management and practice level. One consultant commented that to work together with mental health–substance use problems would be too costly. Furthermore, the consultant believed it would create 'too much work'! Consequently, there is a long way to go – but a driving force to succeed exists.

Obtaining in-depth and knowledgeable text is difficult in new areas of change. One needs to be motivated to trawl a broad spectrum of work to develop a sound grounding – the background detail that is needed to build good professional practice. This is a big request of the hard-worked and pressured professional. There are a few excellent mental health–substance use books available. However, this series of six books, of which this is the first, is ground-breaking, in that each presents a much needed text that will introduce the first, but vital, step to the interventions and treatments available for the individual experiencing mental health–substance use concerns and dilemmas.

These books are educational. However, they will make no one an expert! In mental health–substance use, there is a need to initiate, and maintain, education and training. There are key principles and factors we need to bring out and explore. Some we will use – others we will adapt – while others we will reject. Each book is complete. Conversely, each aims to build on the preceding book. However, books *do not* hold all the answers. Nothing does. What is hoped is that the professional will participate in, and collaborate with, each book, progressing through each to the other. Along the way, hopefully, the professional will enhance existing knowledge or develop new concepts to benefit the individual.

The books offer a first step, relevant to the needs of professionals – at practice level or senior service development – in a clear, concise and understandable format. Each book has made full use of boxes, graphs, tables, figures, interactive exercises, self-assessment tools and case studies – where appropriate – to examine and demonstrate the effect mental health–substance use can have on the individual, family, carers and society as a whole.

A deliberate attempt has been made to avoid jargon, and where terminology is used, to offer a clear explanation and understanding. The terminology used in this book is fully explained at the beginning of the book, before the reader commences with the chapters. By placing it there the reader will be able to reference it quickly, if needed. Specific gender is used, as the author feels appropriate. However, unless stated, the use of the male/female gender is interchangeable.

BOOK 2: DEVELOPING SERVICES IN MENTAL HEALTH–SUBSTANCE USE

As mentioned in the preface, the ability to learn and gain new knowledge is the way forward. As professionals we must start with knowledge, and from there we can begin to understand. We commence using our new-found skills, progressing to developing the ability to examine practice, to put concepts together and to make valid judgements. This knowledge is gained through education, training and experience, sometimes enhanced by own life experiences.

Those we offer care to, and their family members, also bring their own knowledge, skills and life experiences, some developed from dealing with ill health. Therefore, in order to make interventions and treatment outcome effective requires mutual understanding and respect.

In the book, primarily we:
➤ explore the comprehensive concerns and dilemmas occurring from, and in, mental health–substance use
➤ inform, develop and educate by sharing knowledge and enhancing expertise in this fast-developing interrelated experience of psychological, physical, social, legal and spiritual need.

The analogy of the house purchaser sums up the approach of the editor and authors when writing this book. Once a property is identified, we need to find out more before we invest further – the first step is to visit the property. On arrival, we quickly grasp a view of the surrounding area, the look of the outside of the house and its grounds. Here we make the decision to enter the property to find out more – or we leave. It is hoped that the reader of this book will stay! The book takes the reader through the front door of mental health–substance use, for some that will be all that is needed, for a decision to be made, and they will proceed to *own the property*. Others will need more information or guidance on the many and diverse approaches to mental health–substance use.

Once we have decided to purchase the property, we look closer and decide what needs updating to meet our needs, what has to be removed, and what needs rebuilding. We decide not to paper over the cracks because this is our property! Providing and developing services in mental health–substance use is not different to this approach. We need to explore what is good about the service provided to date, how this can be improved, what needs revamping, what services, and people, do we need to make the vision work, what must be replaced, and who is best placed to undertake this work effectively.

We look at what is around – we shop for concepts and the functions and facilities that are best for the people we meet, and to whose needs we must relate to. We then plan how we are going to undertake this organisation and when, and how, the changes can be implemented. Once we have a clear idea what is required, we implement – put into practice – the plans.

Then we leave it for years on end untouched! Do we? Should we? Services, like properties, need constant monitoring – they cannot merely be left until we are forced to do something – until they are damaged. Therefore, we must continually monitor and evaluate the service provision. From here, we can develop, build on new services, and update existing services. What we must not forget is that there are people at the end of this change process(es) who need us, the professionals, to make the right decision, for them, at all stages.

We can never know all there is to know. There is always the need to remain open-minded in the approaches to the individual's needs and expectations. It is essential that we are open-minded to the many differing ways we can bring about change, and how we can access new information and knowledge. This applies in terms of both self-learning, and the way we approach interventions with those who are in need of advice and guidance. Each chapter provides direction to further learning, and exploration.

Many learned professionals are willing to share what they know, and listen to the knowledge and advice of others. It is hoped that this fundamental introduction will stimulate us to 'purchase the property', to take full ownership of service delivery, concerns and dilemmas for the individual in need of therapeutic interventions and treatments resulting from problems related to his/her, or someone else's, experiences of mental health–substance use.

From the outset, and at all levels of the health and social care process, the manager and the service developer play a pivotal role in ensuring that care and quality interventions and treatment are achieved. What he/she does at that point depends on his/her knowledge, skills and attitudes. Moreover, it requires that these professionals acknowledge their responsibility to use the knowledge of others when providing the best services for the individual experiencing mental health–substance use problems.

To have knowledge and skill, there is a need to know something about the bigger picture and how that fits into the care of the individual, the family and carers on whose lives it will impact. Once we have that information, there is a need to know how to develop these services so as to maximise the intervention. To fully comprehend, and understand, we then need to appreciate what it is like to be on the receiving end of these interventions – only then can a service be developed to address the individuals' needs.

It is one thing to look after the person with the physical, psychological, emotional, spiritual, social and/or legal problems, but there is an inbuilt need to care for the professional who provides that care. By so doing, the good manager has a direct impact on the professionalism of the person providing the intervention.

This book is primarily for the student, junior and senior manager, administrator, and service developer and commissioners. In addition, the ward manager, team manager, and clinician need to have some knowledge of how services come to being, the impact that has on them, what steps he/she can take to improve the lot for him/herself, others and the individual with the health issue. Therefore, this book has relevance to educators and students as well as those providing and developing services in mental health–substance use that focus on the therapeutic relationship (*see* Book 4, Chapter 2).

Senior managers, service developers, and ward-based professionals need to understand the experiences of the individual and family, and accept their individual needs without judgement. Moreover, there is a need to understand what factors, beyond the mental health–substance use concerns and dilemmas that affect their lives and influence the services they need. This cannot be achieved without involving the individual, the family and the carers, who also experience the concerns and dilemmas associated with mental health–substance use, at all levels of the service development, provision and ongoing practices.

There is a trend towards 'targets'. This appears to have taken over from the care of the individual to the extent that meeting the target(s) takes precedence. A recent number of experiences highlighted this fact for the author while on an orthopaedic ward. The professionals involved in the care were excellent. However, the demands for bed space precluded care of the individual. The responsibility to 'clear beds', lay heavily with the ward professionals, who had a number of people in a cramped space waiting for the 'bed'. This meant that the individual could progress to theatre without knowing where he/she would be. The anxiety this provoked to vacate beds was the primary focus – taking care away from the individual. Hence, we employ the ward-based professional to 'bed care' and not 'individual care'. When planning services, the good manager ensures that the ward-based professional is employed to do what he/she is best trained to do – otherwise 'care' becomes counter-productive.

In Chapter 2, we look back at the history related to policy in mental health and substance use. By looking back, we can examine where we need to go. Epidemiology issues need to be addressed in that such data helps us to formulate concepts and approaches to a given group of people, this is demonstrated in Chapter 3. Tom Dodd and Ann Gory describe their work in relation to the National Mental Health Development Unit in England in Chapter 4, then Hermine Graham takes this forward to look specifically at developing integrated services in Chapter 5. Gary Croton, in Chapter 6, describes the actions taken in Australia to developing a rural service. He explains the importance of education and training, why this needs to be a concerted effort, and why there is a need to allow time to develop and bring in specific services.

Not all interventions and treatments need to be ward based; indeed a great deal can be undertaken in the community with the correct planning and resources (Chapter 7). Moreover, there is a need to be creative when looking at and developing these services – one size does not fit all. Therefore, we need to pick the best, develop the new and remove the impractical. Failing to consider this leads to ineffective services and poor treatment outcome(s). It is not the fault of the professional, or the individual, it is the fault of poor planning and management. Guidelines are a helpful means of exploring the needs within mental health and substance use (Chapter 8). However, they must be fluid to leave room to address specific individual and service needs and provision. Mandy Barrett, Chapter 9, offers guidance on strategy development, policies and procedure, as a means of learning more, and developing new concepts, for those new to this area of expertise.

Chapters 10, 11 and 12 concentrate on the specific needs of the professional on whom we rely totally when bringing about effective service improvements and developments. The good manager is aware of the demands placed on the professional, and is keen to identify areas of concern and stress. It is imperative that service developers and managers take the professional with them; to do this there needs to be good, effective, quality team work, and good communication practices, without which we fail!

When developing new services, or reorganising services, there is a primary need to explore what is relevant and important to the individual, the family and the carers. Often forgotten or excluded areas are spirituality (Chapter 13) and sexuality (Chapter 14). Spirituality is not about religion but about the individual, where he/she is in society and, just as important, within him/herself. Likewise, sexuality is an individual experience. It is not merely about sexual orientation but about how we as individuals see ourselves and our place in society. It is not the role of the professional, manager or service developer to direct or dictate, not to sit in judgement, but to recognise that each is an individual – each has his/her own rights – we are there to offer intervention and treatment to the best of our abilities.

To conclude, Chapter 15 (Nicola Glover) emphasises the need to acknowledge the rights of the individual to be treated as a human being, cared for by other human beings, and describes what we need to know about mental health and the legal considerations. While given in a UK framework, much is relevant internationally.

CONCLUSION

Referring to the analogy above, it is hoped that this book is helpful and informative. One would hope that we feel sufficiently stimulated to proceed, having extended and developed this grounding in mental health–substance use. Now that the basics have been explored, we can build upon our knowledge using the 'To learn more', section in each chapter as a guide to further study and knowledge. As one enters each new area of knowledge (each new room), so understanding improves of what is needed – and what is not. With that comes the ability to use an open, non-judgemental and accepting approach to the problems identified by the individual presenting for intervention, treatment, advice or guidance.

Our knowledge and understanding constantly change. The challenge is to remain open and accessible to the knowledge and information that will help each of us provide appropriate therapeutic interventions:

➤ at the appropriate level of expertise
➤ at the appropriate time
➤ at the appropriate level of understanding of the individual, and her/his presenting concerns and dilemmas
➤ at the appropriate cost.

We cannot afford to be cocooned in our belief that all individuals are the same. If this book encourages us to be wise in developing and providing services, then it has achieved its aim. If it helps us to appreciate some of the problems encountered by the individual, family and carers, we have 'purchased the property', and can bring about much-needed changes for the individual experiencing mental health–substance use problems.

If your actions inspire others to dream more, learn more, do more and become more, you are a leader.[3]

REFERENCES

1 Confucius; 551–479 BC. Available at: http://thinkexist.com/quotation/when_it_is_obvious _that_the_goals_cannot_be/202375.html (accessed 9 August 2010).

2 Bloom BS, Hastings T, Madaus G. *Handbook of Formative and Summative Evaluation.* New York, NY: McGraw-Hill; 1971.

3 John Quincy Adams. The sixth president of the United States; 1825–29. Available at: http:// humanresources.about.com/od/workrelationships/a/quotes_leaders.htm (accessed 9 August 2010).

CHAPTER 2

Historical policy context of mental health–substance use

Kevin Morgan and Karim Dar

INTRODUCTION

In the last 20 years or so, mental health–substance use problems and their implications have been well documented. In the US alone, it has been stated that there are 10 million persons with at least one mental health and substance use problem.[1] Studies have indicated that 50%–75% of those attending substance use services also have mental health problems, while mental health service users have rates of 20%–50% for substance use problems.[2]

This chapter explores the historical policy context, from which the current mental health–substance use policy has arisen. The history of mental health–substance use, at least in policy terms, is a short one with the first major policies directly addressing this issue appearing in the 2000s. It is perhaps a mirror image of the familiar clinical situation, with substance use and mental health services each standing back rather unsure of how to address the individual with mental health–substance use problems that has also been evident in the approach to developing dedicated policy. This is likely to be, in part, related to the fact that mental health and substance use services have, in most countries, developed separately, each with their own histories and policy preoccupations.

BOX 2.1 Definitions[3]

Policy
A course or principle of action adopted or proposed by an organisation or individual.

Strategy
A plan designed to achieve a particular long-term aim.

Guideline
A general rule, principle or piece of advice.

It is to give a flavour of these separate histories that we will begin this chapter, initially focusing on substance use policy before looking at mental health policy. Then we will begin to trace the emergence of mental health–substance use as an issue within mental health policy before the arrival of policy directly addressing the issue of mental health–substance use in its own right. We commence with 'policy', and related terminology (*see* Box 2.1).[3]

Despite this apparently simple definition, policy has been a much-contested term.[4,5] What constitutes policy in real terms is not easy to define. While the origin of the word 'policy' relates originally to concepts of the state, the definition used here is more inclusive. In this chapter we use the term in this less formal sense.

THE SUBSTANCE USE POLICY CONTEXT

KEY POINT 2.1

A critical point in the understanding of substance use policy is the distinction between:

- criminal- or legal-related policy, usually aiming to control or prohibit substance use
- health-related policy, which focuses on the management of the harmful effects of substance use.

Historically, the emphasis has been on the first of these approaches, an emphasis that is still apparent.

Alcohol policy

The historical development of alcohol policy is characterised by attempts to control alcohol consumption. In the USA, Massachusetts (1637) ordered that no person shall remain in any tavern 'longer than necessary occasions', while Plymouth Colony, in 1633, prohibited the sale of spirits 'more than 2 pence worth to anyone but strangers just arrived'.[6]

In 1785, Benjamin Rush called the intemperate use of distilled spirits a 'disease', and in 1790, along with his physician colleagues in Philadelphia, sent an appeal to congress to:

> Impose such heavy duties upon all distilled spirits as shall be effective to restrain their intemperate use in the country.[7]

The age of temperance had arrived! In 1826, the American Society for the Promotion of Temperance was founded in Boston. By 1833, there were in the USA, 6000 local temperance societies, with more than one million members. Although originating in the USA, temperance was an international movement and there were close links between temperance reformers in North America, Scandinavia, Australia and the UK.

The role of medicine within temperance became important in Britain and other countries towards the end of the 19th century. In 1894, Norman Kerr, English physician and president of the British Society for the Study of Inebriety declared:

> Drunkenness has generally been regarded as ... a sin, vice or a crime.
> ... [But] there is now a consensus of intelligent opinion that habitual or
> periodic drunkenness is often either a symptom or sequel of disease ...[8]

Doctors like Kerr advocated for a state treatment system for this group of individuals, as at the time the management of this problem was by a fine or imprisonment.

Meanwhile, the US temperance movement progressed in the next two decades to the age of prohibition, the mood of the time captured perfectly by TS Arthur:

> The CURSE is upon us, and there is but one CURE; total abstinence, by
> the help of God, for the individual and prohibition for the State.[9]

In 1843, the first prohibition law was passed in the state of Oregon. However, Congress actually passed the National Prohibition Act in October 1919. This lasted until December 1933, when Congress repealed the Act. However, prohibition did not lead to the changes expected as the demand for alcohol probably continued as before but was now complicated by supplies resulting from the bootleg trade and the circumvention of law, e.g. the inappropriate writing of medical prescriptions for whisky. The consumption of alcohol per capita during prohibition also appeared to have increased compared to the year before.[10]

In recent times, a considerable evidence base has developed examining the relationship between alcohol policies, alcohol consumption and alcohol-related harm.[11–13] It is suggested that three types of policies appear to be most effective in reducing alcohol-related harm.[14]

1 Population-based policies, such as those on taxation, advertising, restriction of hours and days of sale, minimum drinking ages.
2 Problem-directed policies targeted at specific alcohol-related issues, such as drink driving.
3 Interventions directed at individual drinkers, such as primary care-based brief interventions for problematic alcohol consumption.

In general, effectiveness is strong for the:
➤ regulation of physical availability
➤ use of alcohol taxes.[13]

Whereas the impact is generally low for:
➤ educational approaches
➤ public service messages about drinking.[13]

Drugs policy

If the dominant theme in alcohol policy has been the attempt to control alcohol consumption, then in drugs policy it has been largely about prohibition (to varying degrees) and law enforcement.

In 1792, the first prohibition laws against opium were promulgated in China. The punishment decreed for keepers of opium was strangulation! In 1800, Napoleon banned cannabis (hashish) usage among his occupying troops in Egypt noting:

> Habitual drinkers and smokers of this plant lose their reason and are victims of violent delirium.[15]

The critical division in the world of drug policy is between:
- those who continue to believe that the priority should be eradication – or at least reduction – of drug use and availability, whatever the costs
- those who argue that widespread drug use will continue for the foreseeable future and the challenge is to manage this problem as effectively as possible.

This fundamental divide is a source of tension both within and between countries.[16]

In recent years, an important concept in much of substance use policy originating in the health domain has been that of 'harm reduction' (*see* Box 2.2). However, this has often been made into an unnecessarily controversial issue as if there were a contradiction between:
- prevention and treatment
- reducing the adverse health and social consequences of drug use.

Many argue that this is a false dichotomy and that both approaches are compatible and complementary.

BOX 2.2 Harm reduction

Harm reduction is a term used to refer both to a set of general principles used to underpin policies concerning the way societies respond to drug problems, and simultaneously to some specific types of intervention, such as needle and syringe exchange programmes and methadone treatment. The term came into use in 1987, and its principles can be traced back to publications, such as the Rolleston Report (1926), which adopted an approach to opiate dependence that included the possibility of medically maintaining the addict, a principle that was the basis of the British system for some 50 years.[17,18]

A defining feature is the focus on the prevention of drug-related harm rather than the prevention of drug use per se. One widely cited conception of harm reduction distinguishes harm at different levels, and of different types – health, social and economic.[19]

Criticisms of harm reduction include:
- harm reduction keeps addicts 'stuck'
- it encourages drug use
- its underlying intention is to achieve drug law reform and promote the legalisation of drugs.

In terms of the recent prohibitive and law enforcement policy focus, there has been little evidence from studies conducted in various countries that these policies have influenced either the number of drug users, or the percentage of those who are dependent. Moreover, there is an increasing understanding of the limited impact of drug law enforcement on the scale of the drug markets. Despite substantial increases in drug seizures, street drug prices have gone down, with the price for a gram of heroin falling from £70 in 2000, to £54 in 2005. Tougher enforcement should theoretically make illegal drugs more expensive and harder to get. The prices of the principal drugs in the UK have declined for most of the last 10 years and there is no indication that tougher enforcement has succeeded in making drugs less accessible.[16,20]

Moreover, it is suggested that these enforcement policies have had a number of unintended consequences:[21]

➤ The development of a huge criminal black market that operates to move prohibited substances from producers to consumers: the financial incentives to enter this market are enormous and there is no shortage of criminals competing to claw out a share of a market in which, hundred-fold increases in price from production to retail are not uncommon.

➤ Policy displacement, whereby public health and the health agenda in general become forced into the background in the face of the preoccupation with the enforcement and legal approaches to the problem.

➤ Geographical displacement: called the 'balloon effect' because squeezing (tighter controls) one place produces a swelling (increase) in another.

Case study 2.1: cannabis, mental health and the politics of policy
Cannabis is the illicit drug with the highest mass consumption. In 2009, the UK reclassified cannabis from Class C to Class B drug.

Much of the debate around the reclassification of cannabis has focused on its link with mental health problems, particularly schizophrenia. One argument put forth is that cannabis is so dangerous to mental health that it should not have been reclassified, but should be more rigorously controlled.[22]

This argument rests on two premises:

1 That cannabis use causes mental health problems
Research indicates that heavy and prolonged use of cannabis in those already vulnerable due to genetic or environmental factors can play a role in developing schizophrenia. However, the UK Advisory Council on the Misuse of Drugs concluded that cannabis use increases the lifetime risk of developing schizophrenia by 1%. The majority of cannabis users do not go on to develop mental illness.[23]

2 That strict legal control can reduce the prevalence of cannabis use and therefore, consequent harms
From the perspective of international evidence, data from the USA showed that there were no greater increases in cannabis use or favourable attitudes towards the drug in the states that decriminalised its possession.[24] Data from the

Netherlands suggests that the de-penalisation of cannabis use does not of itself lead to increased use, although the commercial promotion of the drug may have had such an effect.[25]

In October 2009, Professor David Nutt, Chairman, Advisory Council on the Misuse of Drugs (an independent scientific body established by the UK government to provide advice regarding substance use), was sacked by the UK Home Secretary after using a lecture to say that cannabis was less harmful than alcohol and tobacco. He said, '*it had been upgraded from Class C to Class B by the British Government against the Council's advice – for political reasons*.' Professor Nutt attacked what he called the 'artificial' separation of alcohol and tobacco from illegal drugs. He also said that the smoking of cannabis created only a 'relatively small risk' of psychotic illness.

This view was challenged by Professor Robin Murray, Institute of Psychiatry, London, UK, who said that eight studies published since 2002 had shown that the risk of developing schizophrenia, or psychotic symptoms, was higher in those who used cannabis. He said the risk increased in younger cannabis users and those who smoked skunk, the more potent strain of the drug. '*Our evidence was that if you started smoking by the age of 18, then you're about one-and-half times more likely to go psychotic by the time you are 26 . . . If you start by 15 you're four and a half times more likely.*' Professor Murray said 20% of all the people who developed schizophrenia would not do so if people did not smoke cannabis and in particular skunk.[26]

This example highlights two important issues in terms of policy formation

1 That the interpretation of data used to inform policy may differ, even among experts in the field, and that ultimately it is the job of the policymaker to weigh the evidence, expert opinion and wider factors.
2 That policy must pass through the potentially distorting influence of the current political climate and agenda (in this case the UK governmental desire to appear 'tough on drugs') and so may reflect this as much, or more, than the underlying scientific evidence.

THE MENTAL HEALTH POLICY CONTEXT

There can be little doubt that the major theme in mental health policy in the last century has been the move towards community care and the process of the emptying and closing down of the large mental institutions, a process known as deinstitutionalisation.

The extent that this process has influenced the prevalence of mental health–substance use problems is debatable (*see* Mechanic[27] for a discussion about wider social factors associated with homelessness and mental health and/or substance use problems). However, it seems a reasonable and common assumption that increasing the numbers of those with mental illness living in the community and exposed to illicit drugs and alcohol is likely to increase the number of individuals experiencing mental health–substance use problems.[28,29]

Therefore, in view of the importance of this topic in setting the context of mental health policy in general, and the likely direct effect on levels of mental health–substance use problems, this section will begin with an overview of the issue of deinstitutionalisation. We will then trace the emergence of the rising issue of mental health–substance use within policy. Thus, we begin by looking at how mental health policy has perhaps inadvertently increased mental health–substance use before looking at how it has begun to attempt to remedy this situation.

THE ERA OF THE INSTITUTIONS

Mental illness has always existed and there has always been a 'policy', be that expressed through the laws of the day or simply the social mores of the time or region that has informed how this issue has been managed. In earliest times, the family or local community, perhaps involving spiritual or religious authorities, would often deal with matters. With further development and organisation of society came the increasing importance and influence of the state and its legislature in dealing with this issue. An early example, from England, is seen in the Vagabonds and Beggars Act 1494, which states:

> Vagabonds, idle and suspected persons shall be set in the stocks for three days and three nights and shall have none other sustenance than bread and water and then shall be put out of town.[30]

Over the following centuries, much has changed. However, the desire that the mentally unwell or disordered should be 'put out of town' persisted (and, arguably, through prejudice and stigmatisation, persists to his day).[31]

Consequently, institutions to house the mentally ill have existed for centuries. However, the 19th century saw the greatest increase in the numbers of asylums, and the persons treated in them. The UK saw a rise in the numbers 'certified' in asylums from 5000 in 1800, to 100 000 in 1900 (*see* Box 2.3).[32]

BOX 2.3 Factors contributing to increase in institutional care

- An urbanising population more aware of psychotic individuals.
- The rise of commercial and professional society. In the early stages many asylums operated privately and for profit in what has been termed the 'trade in lunacy.'[32]
- Civic values more humane to suffering of individuals previously outcast.
- Increasing numbers of mentally ill (alcoholism, neurosyphilis[33]) and possibly a rise in incidence of schizophrenia.[34]
- At the time, trend towards increased state intervention in social problems, e.g. Poor Law Act, 1834.[35]
- Rise of a more humane attitude to the mentally unwell and of 'moral treatment'.[36]
- Economies of scale, and idea that grouping large numbers together, would be the most effective way of containing or even curing individuals with mental health problems.

- Families desire to have their 'disturbed' relatives accommodated away from social embarrassment.[37]
- Institutions used as instruments of social control to remove 'deviants' from society.[37]

These noble aims were to become gradually overwhelmed by the sheer weight of steadily increasing numbers of people, many with chronic and irreversible conditions, such as neurosyphilis and dementia. At least part of this increase in numbers has been attributed to rising alcoholism because of drastic declines in the price of liquor in the 19th century.[33] The optimism of the early part of the century was to give way to a pervasive pessimism in its later years. Hopes of cure were replaced by eugenic and 'degenerationist' theories that saw insanity as an incurable degenerative disease inherited as part of the sufferers' biology.

Therefore, in the UK, US and much of Europe, the start of the 20th century saw care for the vast majority of those with mental illness provided by an institutionally based system that was often pervaded by a sense of pessimism and little therapeutic hope. Funding became inadequate, staff were often untrained and unskilled and conditions for those in mental institutions became overcrowded and unsanitary. However, the following century would see a dramatic change.

THE ERA OF DEINSTITUTIONALISATION

The last 100 years has seen many great changes in psychiatry and the care of individuals with mental illness. In the social domain, the great sea change throughout much of the world has been the increasing awareness and acceptance that, for the majority of those with mental illness, care and treatment in the community is not only possible but preferable to institutional care (*see* Box 2.4).

BOX 2.4 Factors contributing to decline in institutional care

- Growing public awareness and concern at the inhumane conditions experienced in some mental hospitals.
- Strengthening civil and human rights movements.
- World War I, and the challenge to eugenic view. 'Shell shock' demonstrated clearly that even 'Britain's finest' could be affected by mental illness, thus challenging the role of genetics and refocusing attention on the role of the environment.[32]
- Large number of individuals with mental health problems after World War I/II necessitated increased community treatment and began to demonstrate an increased acknowledgement of its efficacy.[38]
- Desire of nations to reduce spending on mental hospitals.
- Improved pharmacological and psychological treatments.
- Increasing awareness that the consequences of 'institutionalisation' could be as damaging, or worse, than the symptoms of the mental illness itself'.[39]
- Increasing anti-psychiatry movement and challenges to the prevailing psychiatric orthodoxy.[40,41]

The numbers of individuals within mental hospitals fell massively. In the UK in 1950, there were approximately 150 000 such residents. This number had fallen to 30 000 by the 1980s.[42] During the same period, the numbers reduced in the US from approximately 500 000 to 115 000.[27] In Europe, the pace of deinstitutionalisation was slower; all countries (except UK and Ireland) had a higher number of beds in 1970 than in 1950. However, not one European country saw a fall in the number of psychiatric beds between 1970 and 1979.[43]

Given the scale of the change, it is not surprising that deinstitutionalisation has not been without its problems. Apart from the sizeable practical problems involved in developing and providing a network of care for those now living in the community, a number of other consequences have been proposed, including:

➤ increased homelessness in mentally unwell[44]
➤ trans-institutionalisation – the displacement of the mentally unwell from mental institutions to other institutions, such as prison, forensic mental health wards or supported housing facilities[45]
➤ a possible increase in suicide rates.[46]

Where does this leave mental health policy now?

If the period of deinstitutionalisation can be described as 'opening the back door' (of the institutions), then recent mental health policy has firmly switched its focus to 'closing the front door'. In addition to continuing to develop community mental health services, we have seen the appearance of teams taking an ever more proactive role in helping to prevent and reduce rates of admission and support individuals remaining in the community. These have been variously named:

➤ Home Treatment Teams
➤ Assertive Outreach Teams
➤ Crisis Resolution Teams.

Small wonder then, perhaps, that increasing attention should fall upon the individual experiencing mental health–substance use problems for whom it was often not so much a case of closing the front door but attempting to stop the revolving door.

THE EMERGENCE OF THE MENTAL HEALTH–SUBSTANCE USE ISSUE WITHIN MENTAL HEALTH POLICY

The problem of mental health–substance use first began appearing in the scientific literature in the mid 1980s, though a formal recognition had been signalled by the inclusion of categories of drug-induced disorders within the *Diagnostic and Statistical Manual of Mental Disorders*, third edition (DSM-III), published in 1980.[47] However, it was not until the late 1990s that the issue began to filter through into mental health policy documents:

➤ UK – *National Service Framework for Mental Health* [48]
➤ USA – *Mental Health: a report of the Surgeon General* [49]
➤ Australia – *National Mental Health Plan.* [50]

These documents represented little more than an acknowledgement of the mental health–substance use issue and much of the coverage could be summed up by the epithet 'we must try harder'. A sizeable clinical problem was being reflected in only a very small fraction of the policy coverage. Moreover, there was little in the way of operational guidance or clear suggestions as to how services could best be provided for this group or, importantly, resources allocated to enable this.

THE EMERGENCE OF SPECIFIC MENTAL HEALTH–SUBSTANCE USE POLICY

As research continued and the evidence base improved in the field of mental health–substance use, the gradually emerging threads of policy (or, more accurately, references within policy documents) began to coalesce into a specific body of mental health–substance use-focused documentation. In the UK in 2002, the *Dual Diagnosis Good Practice Guide*[51] and *Co-existing Problems of Mental Disorder and Substance Misuse (dual diagnosis): an information manual*[52] were published. In the same year, the US saw the *Report to Congress on the Prevention and Treatment of Co-occurring Substance Abuse Disorders and Mental Disorders*,[53] and the following year Australia produced the state-funded monograph *Comorbid Mental Disorders and Substance Use Disorders: epidemiology, prevention and treatment.*[54]

Barriers to treatment for those with mental health–substance use problems became more clearly elucidated, often a consequence of differences between mental health and substance use services (*see* Box 2.5). Professional began to look closely at how treatment could be most effectively delivered as an accumulating evidence base emerged.[55] Some professionals posited that 'transformation' was needed at every level of organisation, including policy, programme, procedure and practice, and described systems of care through which they believed this could be achieved.[56]

BOX 2.5 Differences between mental health and substance use services[54]

Frequently, mental health and substance abuse services will have differing:
- staffing resources
- philosophies and approaches to treatment
- funding sources and budgets
- training and competencies of staff
- salaries, affecting recruitment and retention of staff
- attitudes to mental health–substance use
- medical involvement
- regulations
- routine evaluation and testing procedures performed
- assertive community outreach capabilities.

The spectrum of problems found in mental health–substance use vary greatly in their nature and degree of severity. Therefore, it can often be difficult to clearly define these problems. Importantly, from a service provision perspective, this can lead to ambiguity and confusion as to which service, mental health or substance use, should be taking the lead responsibility in individual cases. This confusion can contribute to the phenomena of 'falling down the cracks' between services,[57] and has often been cited as an important barrier to care for individuals with mental health–substance use problems.

As a means of addressing this a conceptual framework[1] (sometimes referred to as the quadrants of care or four quadrant model) was proposed, which has been widely accepted and influential throughout much of subsequent policy, albeit in variously modified forms (*see* Figure 2.1).

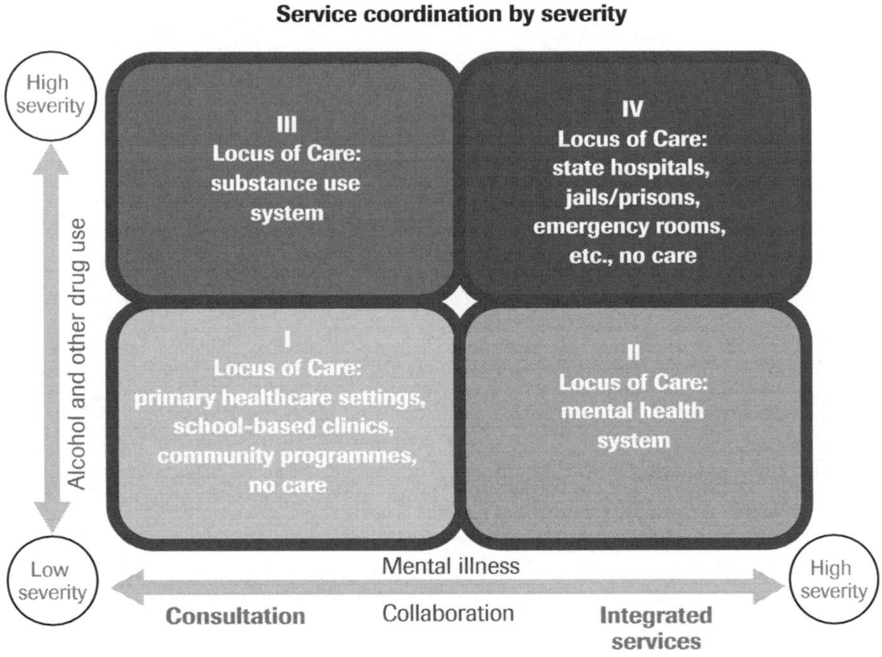

Service coordination by severity

FIGURE 2.1 Mental health–substance use conceptual framework[1]

This allowed for the spectrum of mental health–substance use disorders to be divided into four categories (*see* Figure 2.1). Among the advantages of this model is that it:

➤ is not diagnosis specific but simply relies on dimensions of severity of illness
➤ provides clear guidelines as to which services should take responsibility for management in all scenarios
➤ provides a structure for fostering consultation, collaboration and integration among drug use and mental health services.

In the years following these initial policy documents, much work has been done and progress made. This has been enhanced, and attention and funds concentrated, by the establishment of several national initiatives to act as central sources of information, promote the issue of mental health–substance use, offer guidance to improve service coordination and disseminate best practice. These include the Co-occurring Center of Excellence (USA 2002); the National Comorbidity Initiative (Australia 2003); and the Dual Diagnosis Programme (UK 2009).

RECENT COMMON THEMES IN INTERNATIONAL MENTAL HEALTH–SUBSTANCE USE POLICY AND GUIDELINES

Mainstreaming

The needs of those individuals experiencing substance use problems with severe mental health problems should be able to be met within mainstream mental health services.

Integrated care

➤ There is a consensus regarding the ideal of integrated treatment, particularly for those with more severe illness.

➤ It is acknowledged that this may not be feasible or necessary in all settings and various hybrids might be appropriate depending on the level of need of a given population.

Mental health–substance use is the norm and to be expected in all mental health settings

➤ All services within the mental health or substance use systems should be competent to screen, assess and address mental health–substance use.

➤ Policies and procedures should explicitly acknowledge mental health–substance use and define requirements for addressing the needs of those individuals affected.

'No wrong door'

➤ The integrated system of care must be accessible from multiple points of entry.

➤ The principle that all agencies respond to the individual's needs through either direct services, or linkages to appropriate services, and not by sending the individual from one agency to another.

Individualised and responsive care

➤ There can be no one clinical model of care for people with mental health–substance use problems and each individual's treatment plan must be derived from a careful assessment.

➤ Consideration should be given to, but not limited to, immediate and acute needs, diagnosis, disability, motivation, and stage of readiness for change.

CONCLUSION

This chapter offers an overview of the policy context of mental health–substance use. We have suggested that, in terms of the policy agenda for dealing with substance use, much of the focus and attention has tended to be directed towards the legal and law enforcement efforts that have attempted to control (alcohol) or prohibit (drugs) substance use. Health policy, on the other hand, has enjoyed considerably less prominence.

In mental healthcare, we have described the seismic shift in policy and care of recent times as being the move from institutional care to care in the community. In part relating to this shift towards community care is an increasing awareness of mental health–substance use problems. Consequently, over the last decade and in many parts of the world, specific policy dedicated to addressing this issue has evolved. However, much of this policy has been in the form of guidelines or protocols from interested professional bodies (e.g. Co-occuring Center for Excellence, USA; Royal College of Psychiatrists, UK). There remains a lack of clear policy addressing this issue within the central, national, mainstream of health, mental health or substance use policy. Hence, the political and financial resources necessary to support and drive implementation has largely been missing.

Arguably, therefore, from top down there remains a basic schism illustrated by the non-inclusion of this subject as a major part of national policy. This is further compounded by different attitudes, philosophies and approaches to treatment that still exist between mental health and substance use services. Consequently, the issue of integration and implementation remains largely 'aspiration', based on local areas of good practice – but lacking the clear policy goals and national focus necessary to fully address this issue.

The issue of why policy is not implemented is complex and reasons for the so-called 'policy-implementation gap'[58] are many. These have previously been explored in detail in both general[50] and mental health terms.[60] In relation to mental health–substance use, we would suggest four key central, but interrelated, areas of relevance (*see* Box 2.6).

BOX 2.6 Barriers to implementation of mental health–substance use policy

---

1 Top-down' versus 'bottom-up' difficulties

In terms of 'top-down' issues, there may be a lack of understanding of the roles, views and attitudes of the services and clinicians involved in the delivery of care. From the 'bottom-up' side there may be a need for improved training and education of workers. There may also be ingrained beliefs in these staff regarding their perceived roles and attitudes towards working with people felt to be outside of their usual expertise.[61]

2 Need for clarity of roles between different services and stakeholders

While the principles of 'mainstreaming' and the quadrants of care model are widely accepted the phenomena of falling between the cracks remains all too common. This is compounded by the fact that there are often multiple services involved, including mental health, substance use, criminal justice, housing and social agencies, each with differing philosophies and agendas.

3 Lack of clear operational guidelines and objectives

Policy has tended to be heavy on recommendations and suggestions but light on clear and practically orientated service models or instruction as to how this will be delivered 'on the ground'.

4 Lack of allocated resources and financial drivers

A consequence of a lack of central political will. This is complicated by the frequently different funding streams used to finance the services involved. Local or state versus national funding issues may also influence this, as may general issues concerning the funding of aspects of healthcare through insurance schemes. In the substance use domain (drugs), we would suggest that a disproportionately large amount of attention and resources has been directed towards legal and law enforcement measures with only very limited, if any, effect. This has been at the cost of health-based approaches, for which the evidence base is considerably stronger.

While policy is beginning to appear relating to mental health–substance use in ever more specialised settings,[62,63] there remains a considerable need to develop the capabilities of generic mental health and substance use services to deal with this issue. Until there is a common will to understand and resolve the issues noted above problems are likely to remain. Inherent contradictions that began with the historically fragmented policy development are still apparent today in the way many services are organised and delivered. There are increasing examples of good practice, but until these are more consistently applied the hope of 'integration', in every sense, might be a dream left unfulfilled for several more years to come.

REFERENCES

1 National Association of State Mental Health Program Directors (NASMHPD) and National Association of State Alcohol and Drug Abuse Directors (NASADAD). *National Dialogue on Co-occurring Mental Health and Substance Abuse Disorders.* Alexandria, VA, and Washington, DC: NASMHPD/NASADAD; 1999. Available at: www.nasmhpd.org/general_files/publications/NASADAD%20NASMHPD%20PUBS/National%20Dialogue.pdf (accessed 26 May 2010).

2 Center for Substance Abuse Treatment. *Substance Abuse Treatment for Persons with Co-occurring Disorders. Treatment Improvement Protocol (TIP) Series 42.* Department of Health and Human Services. Publication No. (SMA) 05–3992. Rockville, MD: Substance Abuse and Mental Health Services Administration; 2005.

3 *Concise Oxford Dictionary.* 10th ed. Oxford: Oxford University Press; 1999.

4 Colebatch H. *Policy.* 2nd ed. Buckingham: Open University Press; 2002.

5 Hudson J, Lowe S. *Understanding the Policy Process.* Bristol: Policy Press; 2004.

6 Cherrington E. *The Evolution of Prohibition in the United States of America.* Westerville, OH: American Issue Press; 1920. p. 18.

7 Benjamin Rush. As cited in: Crafts WF, Leitch M, Letch MW. *Intoxicating Drinks and Drugs in All Lands and Times.* Washington, DC: The International Reform Bureau; 1909. p. 9.

8 Norman Kerr. As cited in: Roueche B. *The Neutral Spirit: a portrait of alcohol.* Boston, MA: Little, Brown & Co.; 1960. pp. 107–8.

9 Arthur TS. *Grappling with the Monster; or the Curse and the Cure of Strong Drink.* New York, NY: JW Lovell & Co.; 1877.

10 Tillitt MH. *The Price of Prohibition.* New York, NY: Harlehurst, Brace & Co.; 1932. pp. 35–6.

11 Bruun K, Edwards G, Lumio M, *et al. Alcohol Control Policies in Public Health Perspective.* Helsinki: Finnish Foundation for Alcohol Studies; 1975.

12 Edwards G, Anderson P, Babor TF, *et al. Alcohol Policy and the Public Good.* New York, NY: Open University Press; 1994.

13 Babor TF, Caetauo R, Casswell S, *et al. Alcohol: no ordinary commodity. Research and public policy.* Oxford: Open University Press; 2003.

14 Anderson P. Addiction and alcohol use disorders. In: Knapp M, McDaid D, Mossialos E,

Thornicroft G, editors. *Mental Health Policy and Practice across Europe.* Maidenhead: Open University Press; 2007.

15 Ernest A. *Marihuana: the first twelve thousand years.* New York, NY: Plenum Press; 1980.

16 Roberts M, Bewley-Taylor D, Trace M. *Facing the Future: the challenge for national and international drug policy.* Report 6. The Beckley Foundation Drug Policy Programme; 2005. Available at: www.beckleyfoundation.org/pdf/Report_06.pdf (accessed 26 May 2010).

17 Stimson GV, Oppenheimer E. *Heroin Addiction: treatment and control in Britain.* London: Tavistock; 1982.

18 Strang J, Gossop M. Heroin prescribing in the British system: a historical review. *Eur Addict Res.* 1996; **2**: 185–93.

19 Newcombe R. The reduction of drug-related harm: a conceptual framework for theory, practice and research. In: O'Hare PA, Newcombe R, Matthews A, *et al.*, editors. *The Reduction of Drug-related Harm.* London: Routledge; 1992.

20 Reuter P, Stevens A. *An analysis of UK drug policy: a monograph prepared for the UK Drug Policy Commission. 2007.* Available at: www.ukdpc.org.uk/docs%5CUKDPC%20drug%20 policy%20review%20exec%20summary.pdf (accessed 26 May 2010).

21 UNODC. *Making Drug control 'fit for purpose': building on the UNGASS decade.* Report by the Executive Director of the United Nations Office on Drugs and Crime; March 2008. p. 10. Available at: www.unodc.org/documents/commissions/CND-Session51/CND-UNGASS-CRPs/ECN72008CRP17.pdf (accessed 26 May 2010).

22 Phillips M. Reclassify cannabis *upwards. Daily Mail*; 8 January 2004.

23 Advisory Council on the Misuse of Drugs. *Further consideration of the classification of cannabis under the Misuse of Drugs Act 1971.* London: Home Office; 2005.

24 Single E, Christie P, Ali R. The impact of decriminalisation in Australia and the United States. *J Public Health Policy.* 2000; **21**: 157–86.

25 MacCoun R, Reuter P. Evaluating alternative cannabis regimes. *Br J Psychiatry.* 2001; **178**: 123–8.

26 BBC Online. *Sacked adviser urges drugs probe.* 19 November 2009. Available at: news.bbc.co.uk/1/hi/uk/8366466.stm (accessed 26 May 2010).

27 Mechanic D. *Mental Health and Social Policy: beyond managed care.* London: Allyn and Bacon; 2008.

28 Crawford V. *Co-existing Problems of Mental Health and Substance Misuse ('Dual Diagnosis'): a review of relevant literature.* London: Royal College of Psychiatrists; 2001. p. 7.

29 Sirota T, Leo K. Dual diagnosis – North America. In: Phillips P, McKeown O, Sandford T, editors. *Dual Diagnosis: practice in context.* Chichester: Wiley-Blackwell; 2009. p. 200.

30 11 Henry 7 c.2 1494 Vagabonds and Beggars Act. Cited in: Roberts A. *Mental Health History Timeline.* Available at: http://studymore.org.uk/law.htm (accessed 26 May 2010).

31 Thornicroft G. *Shunned: discrimination against people with mental illness.* Oxford: Oxford University Press; 2006.

32 Porter R. *Madness: a brief history.* Oxford: Oxford University Press; 2002.

33 Shorter E. *A Historical Dictionary of Psychiatry.* Oxford: Oxford University Press; 2005. p. 4.

34 Hare E. Schizophrenia as a recent disease. *Br J Psychiatry.* 1998; **153**: 521–31.

35 Pilgrim D, Rogers A. *A Sociology of Mental Illness.* 2nd ed. New York: Open University Press; 1999.

36 Luchins AS. Moral treatment in asylums and general hospitals in 19th century America. *J Psychol.* 1989; **123**: 585–607.

37 Shorter E. The historical development of mental health services in Europe. In: Knapp M,

McDaid D, Mossialos E, *et al.*, editors. *Mental Health Policy and Practice across Europe.* Buckingham: Open University Press; 2007.

38 Grob G. *From Asylum to Community: mental health policy in modern America.* Oxford: Princeton University Press; 1991.

39 Goffman E. *Asylums: essays on the social situation of mental patients and other inmates.* Port Moody, BC: Anchor; 1961.

40 Szasz T. *The Myth of Mental Illness: foundations of a theory of personal conduct.* New York, NY: Hoeber-Harper; 1961.

41 Foucault M. *Madness and Civilization: a history of insanity in the age of reason.* New York, NY: Pantheon Books; 1965.

42 Porter R. *A Social History of Madness: stories of the insane.* London: Weidenfeld and Nicholson; 1987.

43 Mangen SP. Psychiatric policies: developments and constraints. In: Mangen SP, editor. *Mental Health Care in the European Community.* London: Croom Helm; 1985.

44 McQuistion HL, Finnerty M, Hirschowitz J, *et al.* Challenges for psychiatry in serving homeless people with psychiatric disorders. *Psychiatr Serv.* 2003; **54**: 669–76.

45 Priebe S, Badesconyi A, Fioritti A, *et al.* Reinstitutionalisation in mental health care: comparison of data on service provision from six European countries. *Br Med J.* 2005; **330**: 123–6.

46 Yoon J, Bruckner TA. Does deinstitutionalization increase suicide? *Health Serv Res.* 2009; **44**: 1385–405.

47 American Psychiatric Association. *Diagnostic and Statistical Manual of Mental Disorders III.* Washington, DC: American Psychiatric Association; 1980.

48 Department of Health. *National Service Framework for Mental Health: modern standards and service models.* 1999. Available at: www.dh.gov.uk/prod_consum_dh/groups/dh_digital assets/@dh/@en/documents/digitalasset/dh_4077209.pdf (accessed 26 May 2010).

49 US Department of Health and Human Services. *Mental Health: a report of the Surgeon General.* Rockville, MD: US Department of Health and Human Services, Substance Abuse and Mental Health Services Administration, Center for Mental Health Services, National Institutes of Health, National Institute of Mental Health; 1999.

50 Australian Health Ministers. *National Mental Health Plan 2003–2008.* Canberra, ACT: Australian Government, 2003.

51 Department of Health. *Mental Health Policy Implementation Guide: dual diagnosis good practice guide.* London: HMSO; 2002. Available at: www.substancemisuserct.co.uk/staff/ documents/dh_4060435.pdf (accessed 26 May 2010).

52 Banerjee S, Clancy C, Crome I, editors. *Co-existing Problems of Mental Disorder and Substance Misuse (dual diagnosis): an information manual. Final report to the Department of Health.* London: Royal College of Psychiatrists; 2001.

53 Substance Abuse and Mental Health Services Administration. *Report to Congress on the Prevention and Treatment of Co-occurring Substance Abuse Disorders and Mental Disorders.* US Department of Health and Human Services; 2002. Available at: www.samhsa.gov/ reports/congress2002/index.html (accessed 26 May 2010).

54 Teesson M, Proudfoot H. *Comorbid Mental Disorders and Substance Use Disorders: epidemiology, prevention and treatment.* Commonwealth of Australia; 2003. Available at: www. health.gov.au/internet/main/publishing.nsf/Content/D588E61C48428185CA256F190004 4A02/$File/mono_comorbid.pdf (accessed 26 May 2010).

55 Drake R, Essock SM, Shaner A, *et al.* Implementing dual diagnosis services for clients with severe mental illness. *Psychiatr Serv.* 2001; **52**: 469–76.

56 Minkoff K, Cline CA. Changing the world: the design and implementation of comprehensive

continuous, integrated systems of care for individuals with co-occurring disorders. *Psychiatr Clin North Am.* 2004; **27**: 727–43.

57 Appleby L. Foreword. In: Department of Health. *Mental Health Policy Implementation Guide: dual diagnosis good practice guide.* London: Department of Health; 2002. Available at: www.substancemisuserct.co.uk/staff/documents/dh_4060435.pdf (accessed 26 May 2010). p. 3.

58 Dunsire A. *Implementation in a Bureaucracy.* Oxford: Martin Robertson; 1978.

59 Gunn LA. Why is implementation so difficult? *Management Services in Government.* 1978; **33**: 169–76.

60 Lester H, Glasby J. *Mental Health Policy and Practice.* Basingstoke: Palgrave Macmillan; 2006.

61 Hughes E, Wanigaratne S, Gournay K, *et al.* Training in dual diagnosis interventions (the COMO Study): a randomised controlled trial. *BMC Psychiatry.* 2008; **8**: 8–12. Available at: www.biomedcentral.com/1471–244X/8/12 (accessed 26 May 2010).

62 Department of Health. *A Guide for the Management of Dual Diagnosis in Prison.* London: Department of Health; 2009. Available at: www.dh.gov.uk/prod_consum_dh/groups/dh_digitalassets/@dh/@en/documents/digitalasset/dh_097694.pdf (accessed 26 May 2010).

63 Department of Health. *Dual Diagnosis in Mental Health Inpatient and Day Hospital Setting.* London: Department of Health; 2006. Available at: www.dh.gov.uk/prod_consum_dh/groups/dh_digitalassets/@dh/@en/documents/digitalasset/dh_062652.pdf (accessed 26 May 2010).

TO LEARN MORE

Australia

- Health policy. Available at: www.health.gov.au/
- Substance misuse policy. Available at: www.ancd.org.au/

UK

- Health policy. Available at: www.dh.gov.uk/
- Substance use policy. Available at: www.nta.nhs.uk/

USA

- Health policy. Available at: www.hhs.gov/
- Mental health and substance use policy and guidelines. Available at: www.samhsa.gov/
- Knapp M, McDaid D, Mossialos E, Thornicroft G, editors. *Mental Health Policy and Practice across Europe.* Maidenhead: McGraw-Hill, Open University Press; 2007. Available at: www.euro.who.int/document/e89814.pdf
- Roberts A. *Mental Health History Timeline.* Available at: http://studymore.org.uk/mhhtim.htm

Epidemiological issues in mental health–substance use: a case for a life course approach to chronic disease epidemiology

Alexander Baldacchino and Ilana B Crome

INTRODUCTION

Mental health and substance use problems are a major public health issue.[1] Pressures on health services and the emergence of competing approaches, such as the organisation of mental health services, have both served to emphasise this burden.

These new pressures on providers of mental health services have resulted in increased attempts to limit the remit of different providers and the development of case-mix in determining the resources made available for interventions.[2] These developments have given rise to a greater focus on diagnostic groupings in some healthcare settings. There has been a tendency in some specialist services to disown the problems of these different groupings (i.e. the seriously mentally ill with problematic substance use within general psychiatric services, and those with personality and other psychiatric disorders within substance use services). This has been further complicated by an assumption that each population belongs to the counterpart service. The result is that people experiencing mental health–substance use problems are left in 'no man's land' or to fall 'between the cracks'.[3]

The prevalence of comorbidity (mental health–substance use) has been reported to be on the increase for the last two decades or more.[4-6] It is suggested that this increasing prevalence may be associated with trends in society as a whole.[7] Examples put forward include:

➤ the increased availability of psychoactive drugs
➤ the individuals involved with mental health services may be more open in admitting substance use
➤ professionals are more alert to the possibility of such use
➤ greater opportunities have been created for previously institutionalised individuals to acquire psychoactive substances and to misuse prescribed substances through the move to care in the community.

Many people reporting substance use have experienced mental health problems at some point in their lives, and many individuals with a mental health problem have a history of past or current substance use. Professionals face a particular challenge from mental health–substance use problems, as they combine to produce greater impairment of function and poorer health outcomes than a single diagnosis alone.[8]

This chapter identifies problems with definitions and other basic methodological considerations when studying the epidemiology of comorbidity. The European co-morbidity epidemiology knowledge base over the last 10 years (2000–2009), will be described. As inconsistencies between studies emerge, they will be discussed, as will the additional research that is needed to examine the specific effect of different drug types and the impact of other factors, such as race and gender. A proposed approach to a life course epidemiological framework in understanding clinically relevant mental health–substance use will be outlined.

METHODOLOGICAL CONSIDERATIONS

Comparisons between different data sets are problematic for many reasons.[9] Some of these reasons are discussed in the following paragraphs.

Conceptual considerations

Considerable confusion and misleading information has arisen from many studies of mental health–substance use because of loose definitions. Confusion has also arisen because, for example, many research groups only vaguely describe specific diagnostic algorithms and the degree to which they consider diagnostic exclusion rules. For a better understanding of mental health–substance use findings, a clear specification is necessary. This is relevant whether none, some or all of the diagnostic exclusions and hierarchies have been considered. Complex sets of symptoms, syndromes, and diagnostic exclusions (as employed by DSM-III-R, DSM-IV and ICD-10) might all affect the resulting mental health–substance use figures, as well as their interpretation.[9]

A further problem with defining, as well as treating, mental health–substance use populations is that, historically, mental health and substance use services have evolved in their own way, using different language and models to inform their service policies and objectives.[10] Additionally, such difficulties may be compounded by different funding streams and fundamental differences in philosophies of care.[11]

Impact of multiple diagnosis and chance association

The type and number of diagnostic classes examined in a study can influence mental health–substance use findings. Simple proportions for mental health–substance use without a description of the specific diagnostic method technique and appropriate statistical analyses (controlling for chance agreement) are practically meaningless. This is because the greater the number of prevalent diagnoses considered in the analysis, the greater the probability of chance association. Studies therefore need to clearly specify what classes of mental disorders are specifically considered and which other axes are included.[9]

Time window for substance use and mental illness and a resolution

Rates for mental health–substance use are dependent on the time-scale for each disorder. Some researchers tend to limit the term mental healt use to current cross-sectional syndromes and disorders, while othe lifetime-ever approach. Only a small number of studies reported specific of cross-sectional diagnosis.[9]

Prevalence figures may be artificially inflated by taking a lifetime overview of a persons mental health–substance use experience, whereas artificially low rates may be generated by adopting a time-limited or 'service year' approach. Findings vary according to whether use or dependence is being assessed over the lifetime, previous year, previous month, or previous week. This aspect can be further complicated by the fact that diagnosis may change over time at an individual level, but moreover the method(s) of assessment and diagnosis may change within a country or scientific community.[10]

Assessment method

The assessment strategy or instrument used to examine mental health–substance use can affect results. For example, a comparison of ICD-10 and the Composite International Diagnostic Interview (CIDI) suggests that standardised instruments reveal two or three times as many diagnoses as the professional would assign in routine diagnostic assessment. This is particularly true for substance use disorders. Although it is not clear which of the diagnoses are valid, it can at least be assumed that the higher mental health–substance use rates of the CIDI cannot be fully explained as invalid. There is some evidence that in the mid 1990s, professionals focused more on the current circumstances of an individual rather than prior history of minor mental health disorders and were more likely to employ implicit hierarchies. Since most professionals were trained at that time in traditional nosological concepts and ICD-9 they were more likely to include in their diagnosis features that might justify a separate diagnosis.[9]

One study[12] suggested that semi-structured diagnostic instruments might be more susceptible to the 'halo effect' than standardised instruments. Another demonstrated that technical modifications can significantly impact on symptom reports, and on the accuracy of dating lifetime episodes of psychiatric disorders;[13] such modifications can include changes to the order in which disorders are assessed, the use of stem questions and memory problems.

Settings

The settings in which studies take place differ, even if at first glance they appear to be similar. Studies of mental health–substance use in one region or location may not reflect the situation in another, especially in the international and European context. For example, it may not be appropriate to compare the rural Highlands in Scotland with inner-city London.

For clinical populations it is necessary to distinguish between general psychiatric and substance use services. For example, in general psychiatric services alcohol and cannabis may be more likely to be encountered as the mental health–substance use

All of these can differ across regions – local, national and international.

Research on 'upstream' factors[17] has been called for, in particular those that operate at a population level, such as housing, income, political systems and social milieu. There are also new opportunities to explore populations in developing countries that have not previously been studied with regard to mental health–substance use. One study, for example, found low rates of mental health–substance use in a traditional Arab community and demonstrated the influence of culture on the assessment and diagnosis of mental health–substance use, as well as on its outcome and service utilisation.[18]

MENTAL HEALTH–SUBSTANCE USE IN SPECIFIC POPULATION GROUPS: A EUROPEAN PERSPECTIVE

We have reviewed the European work in terms of findings from general population studies, studies on substance using populations and studies on psychiatric populations between 2000 and 2009. We describe the studies briefly and seek to draw out issues by focusing on a few studies by way of example (*see* Table 3.1).

TABLE 3.1 General population studies

Survey	Country	Number of subjects	Prevalence of comorbidity	Instruments used
European Study of the Epidemiology of Mental Disorders[19]	France, Germany, Italy, Holland, Spain	21 425	One-year prevalence: 25% alcohol-related problems	Composite International Diagnostic Interview (CIDI)
National Comorbidity Study in Primary Care[20]	UK	4123	Year: 18.7/100 000 Patient Years of Exposure (PYE) in 1993; 36.6/100 000 PYE in 1998	General Practice Research Database (GPRD)
National Household Study of Psychiatric Morbidity[2]	UK	10 108 adults	Lifetime: 22% in nicotine dependent, 30% in alcohol-dependent and 45% in drug-dependent population	Revised Clinical Interview Schedule (CIS-R)
Netherlands Mental Health Survey and Incidence Study[21]	Holland	7076 adults (18–64 years)	Lifetime: 43% of males, 15% of females	CIDI SF-36
Psychiatric Survey on High School Students[22]	Finland	245 (20–24 years)	One month: 39%	Structured Clinical Interview for DSM-IV disorders (SCID)

In the UK-wide National Psychiatric Morbidity Survey,[2] 12% of males and 3%–6% of females had any drug dependence and any current neurotic disorder. People who reported a significant level of neurotic symptoms in the UK study were three times more likely to be drug dependent than those who did not. People who reported a level of neurotic symptoms likely to need treatment were over four times more likely to be drug dependent. Higher total current neurotic symptom scores were associated with a greater likelihood of drug dependence.[23] The prevalence of dependence on any drug was 4%, of which cannabis dependence was reported most often (3%). The prevalence of drug taking in the previous year in 16–64-year-olds had increased from 5% to 12% since 1993. People with drug dependence were likely to be young, male, unmarried, unemployed, in financial difficulty, to be receiving current treatment and to have spoken to a general practitioner about mental health problems or to have used community services, which suggests a degree of mental health–substance use in this population

The National Psychiatric Morbidity Survey[2] also found that people with obsessive–compulsive disorders had high rates of hazardous drinking and alcohol and drug dependence. Neurotic disorders were found to be associated with substance use: while 1% of the population are classified as moderately or severely dependent on alcohol, 2% of those with a neurotic disorder, 5% of those with a phobic disorder, and 6% of those with two or more neurotic disorders are classified as such. Although women were more likely to have a neurotic disorder (20% versus 14%), men with a neurotic disorder were more likely to engage in hazardous drinking, to be dependent on alcohol, to be more heavily dependent on alcohol and to use and be dependent on drugs.[24]

A study of mental health–substance use in primary care in England and Wales, found that the estimated number of mental health substance use cases in the general population rose from 24 226 in 1993 to 39 296 in 1998.[20] The annual period prevalence of mental health substance drug use rose during this time from 18.7/100 000 Patient Years of Exposure (PYE) to 36.6/100 000 PYE; the rate for mental health–substance use increased from 26.1/100 000 PYE to 49.6/100 000 PYE. Although mental health–substance use rose from 10.6/100 000 PYE in 1993 to 16.1/100 000 in 1995, it then fell to 10.8/100 000 PYE in 1998.

Data from the Netherlands Mental Health Survey and Incidence Study (NEMESIS); a psychiatric epidemiological study of a representative sample of 7076 adults from the general population, identified 43% of males and 15% of females with mood disorder as also having a history of substance use problems.[21]

In 245 Finnish young adults taken from the general population, the one-month prevalence for comorbid depression and substance misuse was estimated at 39%.[22]

These studies varied quite widely in terms of subject numbers, time period under investigation, age range, psychiatric and substance use diagnoses, and male/female distribution. For example, the NEMESIS study reported 43% of males and 15% of females as having a mood disorder and lifetime substance use disorder, while the UK-wide National Psychiatric Morbidity Survey demonstrated that 12% of males and 3%–6% of females had any drug dependence and any current neurotic disorder.[23,24]

Institutional studies
Substance using populations

Data on substance use disorders in psychiatric settings are not as readily available as data on psychiatric disorders in drug treatment settings. There is considerable divergence in the populations studied due to methodological issues, as discussed earlier. Of the studies reviewed, the prevalence of psychiatric disorder among drug and alcohol users was higher than among representative community samples (*see* Table 3.2).

Review of European studies points to the diversity of countries in which investigation was undertaken. The UK reported on four studies, Italy on three and Denmark and France on two each. Norway, Finland, Bulgaria, Netherlands, Germany, the Czech Republic, Romania, Austria, Portugal, Spain, Switzerland and Luxembourg each produced one publication.

Not surprisingly, the diagnoses differed, with mood and neurotic disorders being most commonly investigated, followed by psychosis and schizophrenia, personality disorders, and combined disorders. A wide range of instruments was used to diagnose conditions, with little consistency.

In a review of different studies in Germany, Uchtenhagen and Zeiglgänsberger[41] concluded that the most common psychiatric diagnosis among people using drugs was personality disorder, affecting 50%–90%, followed by affective disorder (20%–60%) and psychotic disorders (20%). Between 10% and 50% of people exhibited more than one psychiatric or personality comorbidity disorder.

In reviews of international studies on psychopathology in drug-dependent people, the three main groups of disorders identified were personality disorders (65%–85%), depression and anxiety states (30%–50%) and psychoses (15%).[44,45]

An overview of six studies[16] of individuals treated for substance use in Holland found that antisocial (23%), borderline (18%) and paranoid (10%) personality disorders were particularly prevalent.

Other European studies on populations attending substance use detoxification units and/or residential settings show a wide variety in the prevalence rate and qualification of different types of mental health–substance use. In the Czech Republic, 200 people attending a therapeutic community had a 35% prevalence rate of mental health–substance use (14% personality disorders and 13% depression and neurotic disorders).[31]

In 58 individuals using drugs from a mental health service in Piemonte, Italy, the lifetime prevalence was 58% (22% mood disorders and 21% anxiety, with 16% diagnosed with schizophrenia).[38] In a study of 197 people who use drugs attending a drug addiction unit in Bergamo, a prevalence rate of 73% was established for obsessive–compulsive disorder and one of 67% for depressive illness in opiate-dependent individuals.[37] Another similarly detailed study in Padua established a prevalence of 34% for anxiety disorders, 23% for depressive disorders and 11% for somatoform disorders in 91 people attending a community drug dependence clinic.[34]

Other studies estimated a prevalence rate of 29% in 2180 people attending hospital for drug-related treatment episodes in Finland, of 41%–96% in several studies in Austria, of more than 73% in 596 drug-dependent individuals in Portugal, and of 32% in 380 individuals in a specialised drug treatment service in Luxembourg.[31]

TABLE 3.2 Substance use population studies

Reference	Country	Population	Comorbidity with mental illness	Instruments used	Study methodology
25	Denmark	Heavy cannabis users (n = 1439)	27.5%	Case registers	Lifetime
26, 27, 28	Spain (Barcelona)	Opiate, cocaine and ecstasy users (n = 150)	49% inpatients, 34% outpatients	Psychiatric Research Interview for Substance and Mental Disorders (PRISM) (Spanish) Temperament and Character Inventory (TCI) for Substance Abuse Populations	One year
29	Norway	Polydrug-dependent individuals (n = 287), followed up after six years	90%	Millón Clinical Multiaxial Inventory (MCM-II) CIDI Hopkins Symptom Check List (HSCL–25)	Lifetime
30	Romania (Timis)	Drug and alcohol-dependent individuals (n = 304)	Cumulative: 75% (12% schizophrenia, 12% mixed anxiety and depression, 30% personality disorder [PD])	Case records	Lifetime
31	Austria	Polydrug users attending different centres between 1993 and 2003 (>700)	41%–96%	Review	Lifetime
31	Czech Republic	Polydrug users (n = 200)	Cumulative: 35% (14% PD; 13% depression and neurotic disorders)	Case registers and databases	Current

Reference	Country	Population	Comorbidity with mental illness	Instruments used	Study methodology
31	Finland	Polydrug users (n = 2180)	Cumulative: 29% (psychotic 32%, mood 28%, paranoid ideation 58%)	Case registries and databases	
31	Portugal (Xabregas)	Drug-dependent individuals between 1997 and 2003 (n = 596)	Cumulative: 73% (depression 72%, anxiety 57%, OCD 73%)	SCL-90	Current
32	France	Buprenorphine prescribing service (n = 650)	Cumulative: 30%	Case records	Current
33	International	Opioid dependent (n = 3754)	Cumulative: 78% (42% PD, 31% mood, 8% anxiety)	Meta-analysis (16 studies)	Lifetime
33	Switzerland	Heroin-assisted treatment (n = 85)	Cumulative: 86% (58% PD, 55% mood, 26% anxiety)	SCID	Lifetime
34	Italy (Padua)	Polydrug users (n = 61)	34.4% anxiety, 11.5% somatoform disorders, 4.9% mood disorders	European Addiction Severity Index (Europ-ASI) CIDI	One month
35	UK	Polydrug users (n = 1075)	Cumulative: >33%	Maudsley Addiction Profile (MAP) Brief Psychiatric Rating Scale (BPRS)	Lifetime
36	Denmark (Ringgaarden)	Alcohol-dependent individuals (n = 104)	50% antisocial personality disorder (APD), 30% borderline personality disorder (BPD)	Millen Clinical Multi-axel Inventory (MCMI-II-I)	Current
37	Italy (Bergamo)	Opiate dependent (n = 197)	73% obsessive-compulsive disorder (OCD), 67% depressive illness	Symptom Checklist 90 Revised (SCL-90-R)	Current

(continued)

Reference	Country	Population	Comorbidity with mental illness	Instruments used	Study methodology
38	Italy (Piemonte)	Drug users (n = 58)	22.4% mood, 20.7% anxiety, 15.5% schizophrenia	Case records	Current
39	UK (Bromley)	Polydrug users (n = 74)	Cumulative: 93%	Mini International Neuropsychiatric Interview (MINI)	Current
10	UK (Colchester)	Opioid-dependent individuals (n = 190)	Cumulative: 28.1%	Case records	One year
40	Bulgaria (Sofia/Pleven)	Drug and alcohol-dependent individuals (n = 103)	29.78% (Sofia); 17.30% (Pleven)	Case records multi-city questionnaire SCID	Four years
41	Germany	Polydrug users (n = 200)	50%–90% PD; 20%–60% mood disorders; 20% psychotic disorders		
16	Netherlands	Drug dependent (n = 187)	23% APD; 18% BPD; 10% paranoid personality disorder (PPD)	Personality Diagnostic Questionnaire Revised (PDQR) CMRS Working Alliance Inventory (WAI)	Lifetime
42	UK (London, Sheffield, Birmingham)	Polydrug users and polydrug-dependent individuals (n = 278)	Cumulative: 74.5% in drug and 85.5% in alcohol services (8% psychotic, 37% PD, 68% depression and anxiety)	Case records	One year
43	France (Paris)	Drug-dependent individuals (n = 3422)	Cumulative: 15%	Case records and databases	Current

The prevalence of mental health–substance use individuals is comparatively low in Bulgaria. According to the results of another investigation it is 29.78% for Sofia and 17.93% for Pleven.[40]

Several epidemiological studies of mental health–substance use have been conducted in different populations of individuals, who use substance in Barcelona, including:

➤ opiate-dependent individuals seeking treatment
➤ young opiate- and cocaine-using individuals not seeking treatment
➤ people using recreational 3,4-methylenedioxymethamphetamine (MDMA/ ecstasy), and individuals using substance attending emergency rooms.[26–28,46]

The one-year prevalence of some form of mental health disorder in a drug use inpatient detoxification unit in Barcelona (*see* Table 3.3) was 49% and in an outpatient drug centre it was about 34% presenting with some form of mental health disorder. The one-year prevalence of non-substance use disorders diagnosed can also be found in Table 3.3.

TABLE 3.3 Prevalence (%) of mental health–substance use in different clinical resources of the Institute for Psychiatric Assistance, Mental Health and Drug Addiction, (IAPS–IMAS), Barcelona, Spain

	Emergency room	Drug use ward	General psychiatric ward	Psychiatric hospital	Drug use outpatient centre
Mental health–substance use	11	49	26	12	34
Mood disorders	28	31	47	7	46
Psychosis	20	4	18	61	16
Anxiety disorders	13	4	6	0	16
Personality disorders	31	59	27	13	60
Other disorders	8	2	2	19	21

Around 75% of 210 individuals who use substance (drug and alcohol) attending a psychiatric hospital in Timis County, Romania had at least one mental health condition. Twelve per cent presented with schizophrenia and other psychotic disorders, 28% with affective disorders, 12% with mixed anxiety and depressive disorders and 30% with personality disorders (anankastic, emotionally unstable and histrionic).[30]

In 17 Swiss centres for heroin-assisted treatment, 85 opiate-dependent individuals were assessed at entry using the Structured Clinical Interview for DSM disorders (SCID). The lifetime prevalence of comorbid AXIS I and II disorders was 86%. Most frequently, individuals were diagnosed with personality disorder (58%), mood disorders (55%) and anxiety disorders (26%).[33]

A study conducted in an addiction treatment centre in Ringgaarden, Denmark, identified more than 50% of the 104 subjects, who had severe alcohol problems, as having a diagnosis of antisocial and or passive aggressive personality disorders. Borderline personality disorder was present in 30% of the total cohort.[36]

The Observation of Illegal Drugs and Misuse of Psychotropic Medications (OPPIDUM) survey covered 3422 drug-dependent individuals attending a drug dependence clinic in France. About 15% were prescribed or taking illicit antidepressants and sedatives for psychological problems.[43] Another study of an opiate-dependent cohort attending a buprenorphine prescribing service found that 30% of the participants had confirmed psychiatric problems, with 25% of those questioned having a history of attempted suicide.[32]

In a sample of 287 treatment-seeking substance-dependent individuals in Norway, 90% had a lifetime use, 42% had a combination of substance use and substance induced mental disorder and 5% had a substance induced mental disorder.[29] In a similar study, which looked at 1439 heavy cannabis users who were seeking treatment, 27.5% had at some point been admitted at a psychiatric hospital with disorders unrelated to psychoactive substance use.[25]

The British Comorbidity of Substance Misuse and Mental Illness Collaborative (COSMIC) study found that three-quarters of people in inner-city drug treatment centres suffered from one or more mental disorders: the most common were psychotic disorders (8%), personality disorders (37%), depression and or anxiety disorders (68%).[42]

The National Treatment Outcome Research Study (NTORS) recruited 1,075 adults attending drug treatment programmes, of whom 90% were opiate dependent.[47] Higher levels of psychiatric distress were found for males than for females. Rates for males were: anxiety 32.3%; depression 29.7%; paranoia 26.9%; and psychotism 33.3%. A fifth of all people had received treatment for a psychiatric illness prior to seeking treatment for their drug misuse problems.[35]

One study found an overall rate of mental health–substance use of 45% across a range of five treatment settings (n = 589) in the south London borough of Bromley, ranging from 24% in primary care to 93% among substance use services (n = 74).[39]

A study of two inner-London areas and two cities elsewhere in England found that 32% of substance-using individuals attending drug services had two or more psychiatric disorders, and that 55% of those accessing alcohol services had two or more such disorders.[42,48]

When psychosis in drug use was assessed in Greece, Italy and England, the descriptions of drug use ('opioid', 'drug user', 'polydrug use') and psychosis (schizophrenia, schizophrenia, psychosis) varied, as did the time period of assessment (lifetime, current, one year).[38,42,49] Prevalence spanned 6%, 15% and 8% respectively. Similar issues emerged when depression and neurotic disorders were investigated in Italy, Iceland and Romania.[30,38,50] Current mood and anxiety, lifetime mood and anxiety and lifetime anxiety and depression were examined. One study, found that 23% had mood disorder and 21% anxiety disorder.[38] Another study found that 33% had mood disorder and 65% anxiety disorder,[50] while yet another study reported 12% as having mixed anxiety and depression.[30]

Psychiatric populations

When substance problems in European psychiatric population studies were scrutinised, most studies (7) took place in the UK, followed by France (3), Finland (2) and Denmark. Spain, Ireland, Belgium and Sweden each reported one study (*see* Table 3.4). Service settings included acute psychiatric, inpatient, liaison, and community mental health teams, and others described as 'clinics' and 'services'.

Two French studies reported percentages of lifetime substance use in schizophrenic populations as 43% and 34% respectively.[52,54] However, one study reported 11% current substance use in Croatia,[63] while another study found 7% current and 20% lifetime drug use and 17% current and 40% lifetime alcohol use in schizophrenic populations.[57] Differences in diagnostic groupings and time-frame are apparent.

Even when investigations are carried out in one country, for example the UK, differences can emerge. One study reported one-year prevalence of 36% for substance use in psychosis,[14] yet another study described 19.5% drug use and 11.7% alcohol use in first episode psychosis in the previous year.[64] Settings, services, diagnostic competency and many other factors may account for these variations.

In a specialised psychiatric emergency area within the general emergency department of a general teaching hospital in Barcelona, the prevalence of mental health–substance use in people cared for in the psychiatric emergency room was about 11%. Around 26% of individuals admitted onto the psychiatric ward in a Barcelona general hospital presented with some form of substance use disorder. The one-year prevalence of dual diagnoses among people admitted to a 90-bed psychiatric institute in the outskirts of Barcelona was 12% (*see* Table 3.3).[60]

The prevalence of comorbidity in acute psychiatric services in Ireland was estimated at 26%, following a retrospective study of all admissions between 1996 and 2001.[43] Schizophrenia and other psychoses were found in about 11% and personality disorders diagnosed in 19% of all admissions. A similar study was conducted in Belgium, which estimated that 86% of all 18 920 cases identified and studied between 1996 and 1999 had substance use problems when admitted to psychiatric services. In this situation, 86% of the total cohort were diagnosed with schizophrenia, 43% with personality disorder and 50% with depression. This is a good example of selective admission criteria as a result of locally agreed exclusion and inclusion protocols to decide whom to admit to or discharge from psychiatric services.

A review of studies conducted in Finland prior to 2000, which examined the prevalence of substance use problems in individuals with a diagnosis of major depressive disorder, concluded that the rate varied between 15% and 32% in psychiatric settings.[65] This was followed by a prospective study of 269 patients with a new episode of major depressive disorder enrolled in the Vantaa Depression Major Depressive Disorder Cohort Study, where the prevalence for comorbidity was estimated as 25% of the whole cohort.[58] Also studied were 90 mentally ill, homicidal offenders in Finland, of whom 74% were diagnosed with schizophrenia. Among those who had mental health–substance use (25%) about two-thirds also had a third diagnosis of personality disorder.[59]

In Denmark, the number of individuals in a psychiatric hospital with a secondary drug-related diagnosis increased by 60% between 1995 and 2003. Most of these people were diagnosed with cannabis use or polydrug use problems.[66]

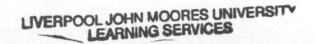

TABLE 3.4 Psychiatric population studies

Reference	Country	Population	Comorbid substance misuse	Instruments used	Temporal framework
51	Sweden (Malmo)	Psychiatric clinics (n = 87)	48.3 %	SCID-I Case records	Lifetime
52	France (Paris)	Schizophrenia (n = 115)	42.7%	CIDI for DSM-III-R Positive and Negative Symptom Scale (PAN NS)	Lifetime
43	Belgium	Admissions to psychiatry services between 1996 and 1999 (n = 18920)	86%	Case records and databases	Lifetime
43	Ireland	Acute psychiatric ward between 1996 and 2001 (n = 1874)	26%	Case records and databases	Current
53	UK (Birmingham)	Psychiatric services (n = 1369)	24%	Clinician Rating Scales for Alcohol and Drug Use (Adapted)	One year
54	France (Paris)	Schizophrenia (n = 105)	34.2%	Chapman Physical Anhedonia Scale PANNS Barratt Impulsivity Scale	Lifetime
55	Denmark	Acute psychiatric services (n = 263)	37.3%	Case records Present State Examination (PSE)	Current
56	France (Bordeaux)	Inpatient unit (n = 127)	Current: 25.2% alcohol, 22.8% cannabis, 2.4% other/ Lifetime: 11.8% alcohol, 11% cannabis	MINI Barratt Impulsivity Scale Physical Anhedonia Scale Sensation Seeking Scale	Current/lifetime

Reference	Country	Population	Comorbid substance misuse	Instruments used	Temporal framework
57	UK (Scotland)	Schizophrenia (n = 316)	One year: 7% drugs, 17% alcohol Lifetime: 20% drugs, 40% alcohol	Operational Checklist for Psychiatric Disorders (OPCRIT) Schedules for Clinical Assessment in Neuropsychiatry (SCAN)	One year/ lifetime
58	Finland (Vantaa)	Major depressive disorder in acute and community psychiatric services (n = 269)	15%–32%	SCAN SCID	Current
59	Finland	Mentally ill homicidal offenders (n = 90)	74%	SCI for DSM-IV	Lifetime
39	UK (London)	Community, forensic and inpatient psychiatric services (n = 589)	26%–45%	MINI	Current
10	UK (Colchester)	Community, forensic and inpatient psychiatric services (n = 590)	16%–34.8%	Case records	One year
60	Spain (Barcelona)	Psychiatric residential services (n = not stated)	11%	PRISM (Spanish)	One year
61	UK (East Dorset)	Community psychiatric services	10% (rehabilitation) 41% (acute wards)	Case records	Current
42	UK (London, Sheffield, Birmingham)	Community mental health teams (n = 282)	44% drug and alcohol use	Case records	One year
62	UK (London)	Psychosis (n = 40)	20% alcohol, 5% drug misuse	South Westminster Substance Misuse Questionnaire Health of the Nation Outcome Scales (HoNOS) Camberwell Assessment of Need Short Appraisal Schedule (CANSAS)	Six months

In France, two cohorts of people with schizophrenic were studied in the Paris region. First, a cohort of 115 established a total use/dependency figure of 42.7%.[52] In the second study, the estimated prevalence of drug abuse/dependency among 105 individuals with confirmed schizophrenia was 34.2%.[54] In another earlier study of the psychiatric population of an inpatient unit in Paris, prevalence of 11% cannabis use/dependence and 11.5% alcohol abuse/dependence was established. The lifetime prevalence was calculated as 25.2% for alcohol, 22.8% for cannabis and 2.4% for other substance disorder.[56]

In a Swedish cohort of 87 individuals attending a psychiatric clinic in Malmo, the lifetime prevalence for substance use was 48.3%.[51]

The COSMIC study,[42] also demonstrated that 44% of individuals in contact with a Community Mental Health Team reported past-year drug use and or harmful alcohol use. Harmful alcohol use was reported by 25% of people and problem drug use by 30%. Drug dependence was identified in 1/7 patients. While acknowledging the limitations of the study, it is clear that mental health–substance use problems should be seen as the core group of mental health services, especially in certain inner-city areas, rather than as a minority group accessing these services.[42]

In a large-scale community survey across mental health treatment services, 24% of a sample of 1369 individuals identified as having severe psychiatric illness had also used alcohol and/or drugs problematically during the past year.[53]

A retrospective matched case control study of a sample of individuals from a mental health trust in Colchester, drawn from adult mental health (n = 400) and drug and alcohol (n = 190) services in 2000, identified a lifetime prevalence of:
- 16% in local Community Mental Health Teams
- 20.6% in a day hospital environment
- 33.3% in an inpatient psychiatric setting
- 28.1% in a community drug and alcohol service
- 34.8% in a criminal justice mental health team setting.[10]

An opportunistic study in the borough of Bromley, London, identified a current comorbidity prevalence of between 19% and 56% among 589 people recruited from Community Mental Health Teams, and inpatient, forensic, substance mis-use and general practitioner services. The prevalence range within psychiatric services, excluding general practice and substance use services was between 26% and 45%.[39]

The Office for Population Censuses and Surveys (OPCS) study found that life-time drug use was reported by 5% of the household sample, but by 10% of those in hospitals, hostels and residential homes.[2] For those experiencing schizophrenia, delusional or schizoaffective disorders the rate was 7%, for those with affective disorders 18%, and for those with neurotic disorders 22%. Of the homeless sample, 28% reported drug use compared to 46% of those attending night-shelters.

One study reported severe mental illness and substance abuse or dependence in 12% of substance use and adult mental health admission (in adult mental health admissions with severe mental illness this rose to 20%), in Eastern Dorset.[61]

In a Scottish community study, 316 individuals with a diagnosis of schizophrenia and 250 controls from the general population, residing within the same postcode area and matched for gender and age, were assessed. Use of drugs and alcohol was assessed using the Schedules for Clinical Assessment in Neuropsychiatry (SCAN). More study individuals than their controls reported problem use of drugs in the past year (22 [7%] v. 5 [2%]) and at some time before then (50 [20%] v. 15 [6%]) and problem use of alcohol in the past year (42 [17%] v. 25 [10%]) but not at some time previously (99 [40%] v. 84 [34%]). The most striking difference between admissions and controls was in tobacco consumption, as 65% of the study cohort were current smokers, compared with 40% of controls.[57]

DISCUSSION

The question of causality: a life course epidemiology perspective

Most of the studies presented above consider the question of causality in a superficial way.[67,68] Current epidemiological exercises in mental health–substance use do not fully tackle the basic methodological processes discussed earlier. This makes comparisons very difficult.

In the meantime, little is known about the precise nature of mental health–substance use in vulnerable groups, such as individuals from different ethnic backgrounds, those who exhibit learning disabilities or chronic pain, and those who utilise non-mainstream services, such as prisoners, street workers/prostitutes and the homeless. Further research needs to look at combining anthropological, ethnographic and health research components in order to help further our knowledge of identifying and supporting vulnerable groups with mental health–substance use conditions. Consideration of children and adolescents and the older population is largely lacking at present.[2,69,70] The implications of this gap in the knowledge base are wide-ranging.

Early screening and identification are more likely to lead to effective treatment interventions, for which there is now steadily accumulating evidence at both ends of the lifespan, as well as in the adult population. This will become highly relevant if epidemiological studies are founded on the principle of a life course approach.[71]

The principal use of the study of epidemiology is to suggest aetiological clues to the condition in question.[72] Over the last few years there has been increasing interest in conceptualising disease aetiology within a life course framework. It is applicable in conditions that experience chronic and relapsing episodes (e.g. mental illness, substance use, oncology, cardiovascular diseases) and equally to a wider notion of health and wellbeing.[73] This approach involves the study of long-term effects on chronic disease risk or physical and social exposures during gestation, childhood, adolescence and young adulthood and in later adult life. It includes studies of the biological, behavioural and psychological pathways that operate across an individual's life course, as well as across generations, to influence the development of chronic conditions (in this case, mental health–substance use). The mere collection of exposure data across the life course is not synonymous with a life course model of disease causation. As a result, few epidemiological studies (and the examples above are no exceptions) explicitly state the temporal ordering of exposure variables and their interrelationships, directly or through intermediary variables, with the outcome measure. This makes discussions around the causality of mental health–substance use very one-dimensional and misguided.

Life course epidemiology of comorbidity reminds us that health at any given point in time is substantially influenced by prior circumstances and that disease processes unfold through a combination of risks operating at multiple levels – ranging from genetic inheritance and psychological vulnerability and/or resilience to social conditions.[74] It is conceptualised into two main stages.

➤ **Stage 1**: 'Aetiologically relevant period'[75] 'critical period'[71] or 'incubation period'.[76]
  — This period might be long, with independent and uncorrelated traumatic factors.
  — It involves multiple causes.
  — It has a cumulative quality that might indicate risk clustering or chains of risks with additive or trigger effects.
  — It contains critical periods when an exposure/stress has lasting and lifelong effects, which may not be modified by later experience.
➤ **Stage 2**: Observable clinical presentation and pathology leading to morbidities and or mortalities.

The time between Stages 1 and 2 is called the latency period.

One can appreciate how this epidemiological exercise will help to identify factors of vulnerability and resilience in mental health–substance use conditions, leading to clearer pathways to causality and ultimate preventive strategies.

Birth cohort data are the ideal means of studying the accumulation of hazards of various kinds over the life course.[77,78] Birth cohort studies, however, are scarce and the members of even the oldest studies have not yet aged to the period in life, early old age, when morbidity and premature mortality become common. Consequently, for the present, any investigation of life course influences on health in the high morbidity and high mortality age groups must use a different type of study design. The study design that shows most promise is known as combining archived survey, which uses records and other databases that can be cross-linked with retrospective data collected by a validated interview method.[79]

Life course epidemiology in mental health–substance use will also allow investigators to start testing for inter-generational exposure disease association. Maternal and paternal vulnerabilities such as lifestyle factors, long-term adverse socio-economic circumstances, growth and childhood will add another layer of rich information to the epidemiology of mental health–substance use conditions.[80–82]

This life course perspective is even now being mooted as a potential model to explain social inequalities in health, since it allows understanding in variations in health and disease of populations over time, across countries and between social groups.[83]

While obtaining adequate exposure measures across the life course may be problematic, so is the analysis of such a large and complex dataset. It is possible that current underused techniques, such as structural equation modelling, path analysis, G-estimation and multilevel modelling, or newer techniques will evolve to help us to understand mental health–substance use conditions and their epidemiology.[84]

Comorbidity epidemiology and clinical relevance

A life course epidemiological approach to mental health–substance use encourages integration of biological and social factors. It also acknowledges the temporal relationships between risk factors and meaningful exposures.

People with mental health–substance use conditions suffer from health conditions or impairments that may result from, or in, a devalued sense of themselves. This might be due to their life circumstances, for example homelessness, poverty, imprisonment, family conflict or breakdown, or social isolation. It might be related to their behaviour (e.g. substance misuse or criminal behaviour), their status (e.g. being older, a refugee or immigrant or a victim of abuse), or a sense of devalued personal quality (e.g. low self-esteem or decreased functional life skills to enable independent living).[85]

In comparison to people with a single diagnosis, those who present with mental health–substance use problems may have a variety of exacerbated problems, and have a poorer prognosis. The most consistent predictor of a poor treatment outcome for individuals in treatment for substance use is the presence of psychopathology.[86,87] Similarly, substance use is a predictor of poor treatment outcome for people with mental health problems.[88] Research evidence suggests that drug treatment outcomes improve if mental disorders are treated.[89]

There are four main domains in which mental health–substance use becomes an important and relevant clinical condition.

1 Self-harm, suicide and early mortality

It is reported that the individuals with mental health–substance use problems have an increased likelihood of suicide.[90] Self-destructive and antisocial behaviours may develop in extreme situations, leading to homelessness, disengagement from the family and community and the development of high–risk behaviours, such as offending, intravenous drug use, needle sharing, suicide attempts, unsafe sex, and binge consumption.[91] There is also an increased risk of early mortality.[92]

2 Psychological problems

Mental health–substance use conditions tend to present with more severe mental health problems. Indeed, admission rates among people in inner London were double those of people with psychosis alone.[14] Increases in impulsive, aggressive and disinhibited behaviours, and increases in anxiety, depression and self-harm, have been associated with the mental health–substance use problems.[92] Social problems, difficulties with activities of daily living, worsening physical health and significant legal and financial difficulties may also result.[93]

3 General consequences

A variety of negative outcomes are associated with mental health–substance use, including higher rates of relapse and rehospitalisation.[94,95] In the largest longitudinal follow-up studies, people with substance-induced mental disorders at baseline were more likely to have been re-hospitalised than those individuals with a single diagnosis, and had the most severe alcohol and drug-related impairment.[96] There was also a higher rate of hospitalisation, violence, arrest and imprisonment, homelessness, poorer housing stability, and serious infections like HIV and hepatitis.[97–102] There is also the likelihood of less compliance with medication and other interventions, and thus more likely to slip through care.

4 Social and economic cost

Those with a mental health–substance use problems place a heavy burden on the range of public services.[103] This is particularly the case if individuals present with a combination of problems, for example severe psychotic disorder and substance use, and a constellation of social issues (homelessness, poverty, criminality, unemployment, marginalisation). A particular strain is placed on acute psychiatric services.[104,105] The costs of providing treatment for the individual experiencing mental health–substance use problems are disproportionately higher than for the individual experiencing psychiatric disorders alone. Poor social outcomes further impact on carers and the family, and on the wider community.[105]

CONCLUSION

The epidemiology of mental health–substance use is currently one-dimensional, as demonstrated by the European studies. A life-course approach, utilising cross-linkage techniques within an appropriate analytic framework, would help to identify the pathways by which risk factors contribute to the aetiology of comorbid conditions. This would help to deliver a more unified treatment and prevention strategy, which is currently lacking due to methodological limitations in current studies and or inadequate conceptual frameworks that do not mirror real-life scenarios.

KEY POINTS 3.1

- Current epidemiological study designs exhibit significant mental health–substance use populations in both substance misuse and psychiatric populations.
- The study methodology used in the epidemiology of mental health–substance use problems are limited by poor internal and external validity, which will limit the interpretation of the results, obtained.
- A life course methodology currently used in other chronic and relapsing conditions, together with effective cross-linkage techniques will help identify, in a meaningful and therapeutic manner, the extent, and contributory factors present in a population with mental health–substance use problems.

ACKNOWLEDGEMENT

The authors would like to thank Corrina Knight for her invaluable administrative support in finalising this chapter.

REFERENCES

1 The World Bank. *World Development Report 1993: investing in health – world development indicators.* New York, NY: Oxford University Press; 1993.

2 Farrell M, Howes S, Taylor C, *et al.* Substance misuse and psychiatric comorbidity: An over-view of the OPCS National Psychiatric Morbidity Survey. *Int Rev Psychiatry.* 2003; **15**: 43–9.

3 Abou-Saleh MT, editor. Dual diagnosis of substance misuse and psychiatric disorders: a US–UK perspective. *Acta Neuropsychiatrica.* 2004; **16**: 1–53.

4 Cuffel BJ. Prevalence estimates of substance abuse in schizophrenia and their correlates. *J Nerv Ment Dis.* 1992; **180**: 589–92.

5 Druglink. Dual diagnosis: factsheet no. 17. *Druglink.* 1996; **11**: 14–15.

6 Crawford V, Crome IB, Clancy C, editors. Co-existing problems of mental health and substance misuse (dual diagnosis): a literature review. *Drugs: Educ Prev Pol.* 2003; **10**: S1–74.

7 Franey C, Quirk A. *Dual Diagnosis: executive summary number 51.* London: The Centre for Research on Drugs and Health Behaviour; 1996.

8 Holland M. How substance use affects people with mental illness. *Nurs Times.* 1999; **95**: 46–8.

9 Wittchen HU. Critical issues in the evaluation of comorbidity of psychiatric disorders. *Br J Psychiatry.* 1996; **168**: 9–16.

10 Todd J, Green G, Harrison M, *et al.* Defining dual diagnosis of mental illness and substance misuse: some methodological issues. *J Psychiatr Ment Health Nurs.* 2004; **11**: 48–54.

11 Lehman A, Dixon L. *Double Jeopardy: chronic mental illness and substance use disorders.* Switzerland: Harwood Academic Publishers; 1995.

12 Francis A, Widinger T, Fyer MR. The influence of classification methods on comorbidity. In: Maser JD, Cloninger CR, editors. *Comorbidity of Mood and Anxiety Disorders.* Washington, DC: American Psychiatric Publishing; 1990. pp. 41–60.

13 Kessler RC, McGonagle KA, Zhao S, *et al.* Lifetime and 12-month prevalence of DSM-III-R psychiatric disorders in the United States: results from the National Comorbidity Study. *Arch Gen Psychiatry.* 1994; **51**: 8–19.

14 Menezes PR, Johnson S, Thornicroft G, *et al.* Drug and alcohol problems among individuals with severe mental illness in south London. *Br J Psychiatry.* 1996; **168**: 612–19.

15 Brown S. Substance misuse in a chronic psychosis population. *Psychiatr Bull.* 1998; **22**: 595–8.

16 Verheul R, van den Brink W, Hartgers C. Personality disorders predict relapse in alcoholic patients. *Addict Behav.* 1998. **23**: 869–82.

17 Abou-Saleh MT, Janca A. The epidemiology of substance misuse and comorbid psychiatric disorders. *Acta Neuropsychiatr* 2004; **16**: 3–8.

18 Abou-Saleh MT. Al Ain community psychiatric survey: prevalence and sociodemographic correlates. *Soc Psychiatry Psychiatr Epidemiol.* 2001: **36**: 20–8.

19 Alonso J, Angermeyer MC, Bernert S, *et al.* Sampling and methods of the European Study of the Epidemiology of Mental Disorders (ESEMeD) project. *Acta Psychiatr Scand Suppl.* 2004; **420**: 8–20.

20 Frisher M, Collins J, Millson D, *et al.* Prevalence of comorbid psychiatric illness and substance abuse in primary care in England and Wales. *J Epidemiol Community Health.* 2004; **58**: 1036–41.

21 de Graaf R, Bilj RV, Spijker J, *et al.* Temporal sequencing of lifetime mood disorder in relation to comorbid anxiety and substance use disorders: findings from the Netherlands Mental Health Survey and Incidence Study. *Soc Psychiatry Psychiatr Epidemiol.* 2003; **28**: 1–11.

22 Aalto-Setala T, Marttunen M, Tuvlio-Henriksson A, *et al.* One month prevalence of depression and other DSM IV disorders amongst young adults. *Psychol Med.* 2001; **36**: 20–8.

23 Coulthard M, Farrell M, Singleton N, *et al. Tobacco, Alcohol and Drug Use and Mental*

Health. Available at: www.statistics.gov.uk/downloads/theme_health/Tobacco_etc_v2.pdf (accessed 3 June 2010).

24 Singleton N, Bumpstead R, O'Brien M, *et al. Psychiatric Morbidity Among Adults Living in Private Households, 2000*. Available at: www.statistics.gov.uk/downloads/theme_health/psychmorb.pdf (accessed 3 June 2010).

25 Arendt M, Munk-Jorgensen P. Heavy cannabis users seeking treatment: prevalence of psychiatric disorders. *Soc Psychiatry Psychiatr Epidemiol*. 2004; **39**: 97–105.

26 Astals M, Torrens M, Domingo-Salvany A, *et al.* Comorbidity in opioid addicts in methadone maintenance treatment: preliminary results [Paper presented at conference]. *5th Conference of the European Opiate Addiction Treatment Association*. Oslo; 2002.

27 Ginés JM, Fonseca F, Poudevida S, *et al.* Psychiatric comorbidity in ecstasy users: a one year follow-up controlled study. *Eur Psychiatry*. 2004; **19**: S158–9

28 Rodríguez-Llera MC, Domingo-Salvany A, Brugal MT, *et al.* [Prevalence of dual diagnosis in young consumers of heroin: preliminary results] [Spanish]. *Gaceta Sanitaria*. 2002; **16**: 104.

29 Bakken K, Landheim AS, Vaglum P. Primary and secondary substance misusers: do they differ in substance-induced and substance-independent mental disorders? *Alcohol Alcohol*. 2003; **38**: 54–9.

30 Enatescu VR, Dehelean L. Psychiatric comorbidity in patients with substance misuse in Romania. In: Baldacchino A, Corkery J, editors. *Comorbidity: perspectives across Europe: ECCAS monograph no. 4*. London: European Collaborative Centre in Addiction Services; 2006. pp. 221–34.

31 European Monitoring Centre for Drugs and Drug Addiction (EMCDDA). *Comorbidity: drug use and mental disorders – drugs in focus 14*. Available at: www.emcdda.europa.eu/html.cfm/index36329EN.html (accessed 3 June 2010).

32 Fihma A, Henrion R, Lowenstein W, *et al.* [Two-year follow-up of an opioid-user cohort treated with high-dose buprenorphine (Subutex)] [French]. *Annales de Medicine Interne*. 2001; **152**: IS26–36.

33 Frei A, Rehm J. [Comorbidity: psychiatric disorder of opiate addicts at entry into heroin assisted treatment] [German]. *Psychiatr Prax*. 2002; **29**: 251–7.

34 di Furia L, Pizza M, Rampazzo L, *et al.* Comorbidity in Padua. In: Baldacchino A, Corkery J, editors. *Comorbidity: perspectives across Europe – ECCAS monograph no. 4*. London: European Collaborative Centre in Addiction Services; 2006. pp. 186–98.

35 Gossop M, Marsden J, Stewart D, *et al.* The National Treatment Outcome Research Study (NTORS): 4–5 year follow-up results. *Addiction*, 2003; **98**: 291–303.

36 Nielsen P, Rojskaer S. [Dual disorders among alcohol addicted inpatient clients] [Norwegian]. *Nordisk Alkohol-og Narkotikatidsskrift*. 2002; **19**: 123–37.

37 Riglietta M, Beato E, Colombo L, *et al.* Drugs and psychosis in Italy: historical overview and recent perspectives. In: Baldacchino A, Corkery J, editors. *Comorbidity: perspectives across Europe – ECCAS monograph no. 4*. London: European Collaborative Centre in Addiction Services; 2006.

38 Siliquini R, Zeppegno P, Faggiano F. [Psychiatric pathology and consumption of substances: preliminary description of the cases of a case-control study] [Italian]. In: Faggiano F, editor. *OED Piemonte: rapporto 2002*. Turin: Osservatorio Epidemiologico Dipendenze; 2002.

39 Strathdee G, Manning V, Best D. *Dual Diagnosis in a Primary Care Group (PCG): a step-by-step epidemiological needs assessment and design of a training and service response model – research summaries for providers and commissioners RS2*. Available at: www.nta.nhs.uk/

publications/documents/nta_dual_diagnosis_primary_care_group_2002_rs2.pdf (accessed 3 June 2010).

40 Toteva S, Rizov A, Tenev V, *et al.* The comorbidity situation in Bulgaria: epidemiological, clinical and therapeutic aspects. In: Baldacchino A, Corkery J, editors. *Comorbidity: perspectives across Europe – ECCAS monograph no. 4.* London: European Collaborative Centre in Addiction Services; 2006. pp. 133–44.

41 Uchtenhagen U, Zieglgänsberger W. [*Addiction Medicine: concepts, strategies and therapeutical management*] [German]. Munich: Urban & Fischer Verlag; 2000.

42 Weaver T, Madden P, Charles V, *et al.* Comorbidity of substance misuse and mental illness in community mental health and substance misuse services. *Br J Psychiatry.* 2003; **183**: 304–13.

43 Wieviorka S. *France: drug situation – report to the EMCDDA by the Reitox National Focal Point.* Lisbon: European Collaborative Centre in Addiction Services; 2003.

44 Fridell M. [*Personality and Drug Addiction: a research overview*] [Swedish]. Stockholm: Centralförbundet för Alkohol-och Narkotikaupplysinings (CAN).

45 Fridell M. [Mental disturbance and drug addiction] [Swedish]. *Psykisk Störda Missbrukare*; **14**: 34–56.

46 Imaz ML, Fonseca F, Ginés JM, *et al.* Dual diagnosis in a general hospital psychiatric emergency [Paper presented at conference]. *VI World Congress of the International Association for Emergency Psychiatry.* Barcelona; 9–12 June 2002.

47 Marsden J, Gossop M, Stewart D, *et al.* Psychiatric symptoms among clients seeking treatment for drug dependence: intake data from the National Treatment Outcome Research Study. *Br J Psychiatry.* 2000; **176**: 285–9.

48 Weaver T, Charles V, Madden P, *et al.* A *Study of the Prevalence and management of Comorbidity Amongst Adult Substance Misuse and Mental Health Treatment Populations: research summaries for providers and commissioners RS1.* Available at: www.nta.nhs.uk/publications/documents/nta_cosmic_survey_2002_rs1.pdf (accessed 3 June 2010).

49 Kokkevi A, Stefanis C. Drug abuse and psychiatric co-morbidity. *Compr Psychiatry.* 1995; **36**: 329–37.

50 Tomasson K, Vaglum P. A nation wide representative sample of treatment seeking alcoholics: a study of psychiatric comorbidity. *Acta Psychiatr Scand.* 1995; **92**: 378–85.

51 Cantor-Graae E, Nordstrom LG, McNeil TF. Substance abuse in schizophrenia: a review of the literature and a study of correlates in Sweden. *Schizophr Res.* 2001; **48**: 69–82.

52 Dervaux A, Laqueille X, Krebs MO. [Schizophrenic disorders and drug addiction] [French]. *Santé Mentale.* 2002; **70**: 16–21.

53 Graham HL, Maslin J, Copello A, *et al.* Drug and alcohol problems amongst individuals with severe mental health problems in an inner city area of the UK. *Soc Psychiatry Psychiatr Epidemiol.* 2001; **36**: 448–55.

54 Gut-Fayand A, Dervaux A, Olle JP, *et al.* Substance abuse in schizophrenia: a common risk factor linked to impulsivity. *Psychiatry Res.* 2001; **102**: 65–101.

55 Hansen SS, Munk-Jorgensen P, Guldbaek B, *et al.* Psychoactive substance use diagnoses among psychiatric in-patients. *Acta Psychiatr Scand.* 2000; **102**: 432–8.

56 Liraud F, Verdoux H. Clinical and prognostic characteristics associated with addictive comorbidity in hospitalised psychiatric patients. *Encephale.* 2000; **26**: 16–23.

57 McCreadie RG. Use of drugs, alcohol and tobacco by people with schizophrenia: case-control study. *Br J Psychiatry.* 2002; **181**: 321–5.

58 Melartin TK, Rystsaelae HJ, Leskelae US, *et al.* Current comorbidity of psychiatric disorders

among DSM-IV major depressive disorder patients in psychiatric care in the Vantaa Depression Study. *J Clin Psychiatry.* 2002; **63**: 126–34.

59 Putkonen A, Kotilainen I, Joyal CC, *et al.* Comorbid personality disorders and substance use disorders of mentally ill homicide offenders: a structured clinical study on dual and triple diagnosis. *Schizophr Bull.* 2004; **30**: 59–72.

60 Torrens M, Fonseca F. Psychiatric comorbidity in drug abusers in Spain. In: Baldacchino A, Corkery J, editors. *Comorbidity: perspectives across Europe – ECCAS monograph no. 4.* London: European Collaborative Centre in Addiction Services; 2006. pp. 236–44.

61 Virgo N, Bennett G, Higgins D, *et al.* The prevalence and characteristics of co-occurring serious mental illness (SMI) and substance abuse or dependence in the patients of adult mental health and addictions services in Eastern Dorset. *J Ment Health.* 2001; **10**: 175–88.

62 Wright S, Gournay, K, Glorney E, *et al.* Dual diagnosis in the suburbs: prevalence, need and inpatient service use. *Soc Psychiatry Psychiatr Epidemiol.* 2000; **35**: 297–304.

63 Kozaric-Kovacic D, Folnegovic-Smalc V, Folnegovic Z, *et al.* Influence of alcoholism on the prognosis of schizophrenic patients. *J Stud Alcohol.* 1995; **56**: 622–7.

64 Cantwell R, Brewin J, Glazebrook C, *et al.* Prevalence of substance misuse in first episode psychosis. *Br J Psychiatry.* 2002; **174**: 150–3.

65 Melartin TK, Isometsa ET. Psychiatric comorbidity of major depressive disorder: a review. *Psychiatrica Fenn* 2000; **31**: 87–100.

66 Reitox National Focal Point. *Denmark: drug situation 2002.* Copenhagen: European Monitoring Centre for Drugs and Drug Addiction; 2004.

67 Beeder AB, Millman RB. Patients with psychopathology. In: Lowinson JH, Ruiz P, Millman RB, *et al.*, editors. *Substance Abuse: a comprehensive textbook.* Baltimore, MA: Williams & Wilkins; 1997. pp. 551–63.

68 Swendsen JD, Merikangas KR. The comorbidity of depression and substance use disorders. *Clin Psychol Rev.* 2000; **20**: 173–89.

69 Crome IB, Bloor R. Substance misuse and psychiatric comorbidity in adolescents. *Curr Opin Psychiatry.* 2005; **18**: 435–9.

70 Crome IB, Crome P. 'At your age, what does it matter? Myths and realities about older people who use substances. *Drugs: Educ Prev and Pol.* 2005; **12**: 343–7.

71 Ben-Shlomo Y, Kuh D. A life course approach to chronic disease epidemiology: conceptual models, empirical challenges and interdisciplinary perspectives. *Int J Epidemiol.* 2002; **31**: 285–93.

72 Morris JN. *Uses of Epidemiology.* New York, NY: Churchill & Livingstone; 1975.

73 Kuh DL, Ben-Shlomo Y. *A Life Course Approach to Chronic Disease Epidemiology: tracing the origins of ill-health from early to adult life.* Oxford: Oxford University Press; 1997.

74 Gilman SE. The life course epidemiology of depression: an invited commentary. *Am J Epidemiol.* 2007; **166**: 1134–7.

75 Rothman KJ. Induction and latent periods. *Am J Epidemiol.* 1981; **114**: 253–9.

76 Armenian HK, Lilienfeld AM. Incubation period of disease. *Epidemiol Rev.* 1983; **5**: 1–15.

77 Kuh DLJ, Wadsworth MEJ, Yusuf EJ. Burden of disability in a post-war birth cohort in the UK. *J Epidemiol Community Health.* 1994; **48**: 262–9.

78 Power C, Matthews S, Manor O. Inequalities in self-rated health: explanations from different stages of life. *Lancet.* 1998; **351**: 1009–14.

79 Blane D, Berney L, Smith GD, *et al.* Reconstructing the life course: health during early old age in a follow-up study based on the Boyd Orr cohort. *Public Health.* 1999; **113**: 117–24.

80 Smith GD, Hart C, Ferrell C. Birthweight of offspring and mortality in the Renfrew and Paisley study: prospective observational study. *Br Med J.* 1997; **315**: 1189–93.

81 Smith GD, Harding S, Rosato M. Relation between infants' birthweight and mothers' mortality: prospective observational study. *Br Med J.* 2000; **320**: 839–40.

82 Smith GD, Whitley E, Gissler M, *et al.* Birth dimensions of offspring, premature births and the mortality of mothers. *Lancet.* 2000; **356**: 2066–7.

83 Leon DA, Johansson M, Rasmussen F. Gestational age and growth rate of fetal mass are inversely associated with systolic blood pressure in young adults: an epidemiologic study of 165,136 Swedish men aged 18 years. *Am J Epidemiol.* 2000; **152**: 597–604.

84 Robins JM, Greenland S. Identifiability and exchangeability for direct and indirect effects. *Epidemiology.* 1992; **3**: 143–55.

85 Molesworth S. Personal communication. 2009.

86 McLellan AT, Luborsky L, Woody GE, *et al.* Predicting response to alcohol and drug abuse treatments: role of psychiatric severity. *Arch Gen Psychiatry.* 1983; **40**: 620–5.

87 Rounsaville BJ, Dolinsky ZS, Babor TF, *et al.* Psychopathology as a predictor of treatment outcome in alcoholics. *Arch Gen Psychiatry.* 1987; **44**: 505–13.

88 Carey MP, Carey KB, Meisler AW. Psychiatric symptoms in mentally ill chemical abusers. *J Nerv Ment Dis.* 1991; **179**: 136–8.

89 Woody GE, McLellan AT, Luborsky L, *et al.* Sociopathy and psychotherapy outcome. *Arch Gen Psychiatry.* 1982; **42**: 1081–6.

90 *Safety First: five-year report of the Department of Health National Confidential Inquiry into suicide and homicide by people with mental illness.*London: Department of Health. Available at: www.dh.gov.uk/assetRoot/04/05/82/43/04058243.pdf (accessed 3 June 2010).

91 Murray D, Ellis R, Enter J, *et al.* Connexions: an integrated service for marginalized young people. *Youth Suicide Prevention Bulletin.* 1999; **3**: 18–22.

92 Evans M, Willey K. *Management of Concurrent Mental Health and Drug and Alcohol Problems: GP drug and alcohol supplement no. 11.* Available at: www.nceta.flinders.edu.au/pdf/GP-Project/GP-Resource-Kit_files/B37-HO3.pdf (accessed 3 June 2010).

93 McDermott F, Pyett P. *Not Welcome Anywhere: people who have both a serious psychiatric disorder and problematic drug or alcohol use, Vol. 1.* Fitzroy, VIC: Victorian Community Managed Mental Health Services; 1993.

94 Swofford C, Kasckow J, Scheller-Gilkey G, *et al.* Substance use: a powerful predictor of relapse in schizophrenia. *Schizophrenia Res.* 1996; **20**: 145–51.

95 Linszen DH, Dingemans PM, Lenior ME. Cannabis abuse and the course of recent-onset schizophrenia. *Arch Gen Psychiatry.* 1994; **51**: 273–9.

96 Boots-Miller BJ, Ribisl KM, Mowbray CT, *et al.* Methods of ensuring high follow-up rates: lessons from a longitudinal study of dual diagnosed participants. *Subst Use Misuse.* 1998; **33**: 2665–85.

97 Haywood TW, Kravitz HM, Grossman LS, *et al.* Predicting the 'revolving door' phenomenon among patients with schizophrenic schizoaffective and affective disorders. *Am J Psychiatry.* 1995; **152**: 856–61.

98 Cuffel BJ, Shumway M, Choulijian TL, *et al.* A longitudinal study of substance use and community violence in schizophrenia. *J Nerv Ment Dis.* 1994; **182**: 704–8.

99 Clark RE, Ricketts SK, McHugo GJ. Legal system involvement and costs for persons in treatment for severe mental illness and substance use disorders. *Psychiatr Serv.* 1999; **50**: 641–7.

100 Caton CLM, Shrout PE, Eagle PF, *et al.* Risk factors for homelessness among schizophrenic men: a case-control study. *Am J Public Health.* 1994; **84**: 265–70.

101 Osher FC, Drake RE, Noordsy DL, *et al.* Correlates and outcomes of alcohol use disorder among rural outpatients with schizophrenia. *J Clin Psychiatry.* 1994; **55**: 109–13.

102 Rosenberg SD, Goodman LA, Osher FC, *et al.* Prevalence of HIV, hepatitis B and hepatitis C in people with severe mental illness. *Am J Public Health.* 2001; **91**: 31–7.

103 Hall W. What have population surveys revealed about substance use disorders and their co-morbidity with other mental disorders? *Drug Alcohol Rev.* 1996; **15**: 157–70.

104 Regier DA, Farmer ME, Rae DS, *et al.* Comorbidity of mental disorders with alcohol and other drug abuse: results from the Epidemiologic Catchment Area (ECA) study. *J Am Med Assoc.* 1990; **264**: 2511–18.

105 Kivlahan DR, Heiman JR, Wright RC, *et al.* Treatment cost and rehospitalisation in schizophrenic outpatients with a history of substance abuse. *Hosp Community Psychiatry.* 1991; **42**: 609–14.

CHAPTER 4

National Mental Health Development Unit: an English perspective

Tom C Dodd and Ann Gorry

The National Mental Health Development Unit is the agency charged with supporting the implementation of mental health policy in England by the Department of Health in collaboration with the National Health Service, local authorities and other major stakeholders. Launched in April 2009, the Unit builds on some of the national work established through the:
➤ Care Services Improvement Partnership (CSIP)
➤ National Institute for Mental Health in England (NIMHE).

The Unit is made up of a number of programmes including the National Dual Diagnosis Programme (*see* To learn more).

In 1999, the Department of Health published a National Service Framework[1] laying down the government's expectations for the next decade around mental health reform, both in terms of treatment models (based on the best evidence available at the time), and how care could be organised to work with defined groups of people. Those individuals who experienced mental health–substance use problems would have their needs met by existing mental health and substance use services. Substantial national funding supported the plan, and the inevitable performance frameworks were put in place to measure regional and local trajectories for the:
➤ numbers of teams
➤ numbers of people engaged and seen by those teams
➤ episodes of treatment
➤ the impact on admissions to acute admission settings.

This is a successful policy that has driven, and financed, system reform at a pace unprecedented in the history of mental healthcare in England. The emergence of Assertive Outreach Teams, Crisis and Home Treatment Teams, and Early Intervention in Psychosis Teams had been critical in realigning care pathways, and in offering more timely interventions matched to assessed need. Those teams, and parts of the system that were driven by specific financial and national performance targets, became priorities for commissioners and reforms became embedded in wider health economies.

Critics of the reforms, argue that the National Service Framework did little to engage carers and families, and was particularly 'secondary care' focused, failing to link more positively to community resources, primary care and third sector organisations, where the majority of people with mental health problems continued to receive their support.

Another 10-year strategy 'Tackling Drugs to Build a Better Britain',[2] identified the need to: '*provide an integrated, effective and efficient response to people with drug and mental health problems*', and created the basis for clearer coherence in the planning and delivery of substance use services across England for statutory and voluntary sector agencies. An updated Drug Strategy was later published,[3] which aimed to reduce the harm that substance use causes society, communities, individuals and the families. Guidelines that prepared professionals (trained and untrained) to support these drugs policies included Models of Care for Substance Misuse Services.[4]

SPECIALIST VERSUS GENERALIST

A number of supplementary guides were published by the Department of Health describing service specifications and expected outcomes for specialist teams.[1,5] There was to be no 'specialisation' for responding to mental health–substance use problems. The national policy was one of mainstreaming, where all parts of the mental health system, and beyond, had a part to play in helping people manage their care. Prevalence rates for people who have mental health–substance use problems means that it is often the norm, not the exception, that people in substance use services, forensic services and acute admission settings experience mental health–substance use problems. High rates are also reported in the caseloads for Community Mental Health Teams, and in primary care settings. It followed then, that any attempt to create a dedicated pathway and teams to work exclusively with the range of mental health and substance use problems, would result in unmanageable referral volumes and would effectively deskill the workforce in other parts of the system. In the absence of targets and trajectories, 'everybody's business' and 'business as usual' became the mantra to drive mental health–substance use policy.

INTEGRATED CARE AND TREATMENT

In 2002, a practice guide was published, which described the principles of integrated treatment, mainstreaming, co-working and local strategic developments.[6] The notion that local determinants, such as a joint needs analysis of local populations would lead to the nature and format of a response to mental health–substance use problems, was implicit.

This guide arrived in the context of a national legacy of separate funding streams for treating substance use (from a philosophical perspective of crime reduction) and mental health problems (from a philosophical perspective of treating illness and relieving distress). Theoretical conflicts and independent treatment target regimes meant that it was rare to find care services organised to work on mental health–substance use problems concurrently, and indeed, this was reflected across those government departments who were responsible for funding these services.

People who found themselves with mental health–substance use problems often felt they fell between the gaps across mental health and substance use services. Each service might insist that the mental health or substance use problems are solved before they can work with the individual. Some services might not see substance use as a health issue in itself, but as a symptom of underlying problems that once treated, would resolve the issues of substance use.[7] Integrated treatment was seen as a preferred solution: *'integrated care appears to confer superior outcomes over serial or parallel treatment'*.[6] However, it was recognised that this was untested in the UK context, and that further research was needed.

SELF-ASSESSMENT EXERCISE 4.1

Time: 10 minutes
What are the probable/possible barriers to implementing integrated care/treatment? Consider social, financial, legal, personal and professional.

The integrated model implied the concurrent provision of both psychiatric and substance use interventions but required the same professionals (untrained and trained), working in a single setting, to provide relevant psychiatric and substance use interventions in a coordinated fashion.[6] However, in summary, one study[8] warned that there are several issues that make implementing an integrated treatment model difficult in this country:
➤ Funding streams are separate and can rarely be combined.
➤ Agency turf issues that may not be able to be resolved.
➤ There are legitimate differences of professional philosophy regarding the best possible treatment.
➤ Professionals may lack the minimum degree of cross-training required for them to work together and understand each other's vocabulary, treatment philosophies and care approaches.
➤ There are multiple, pressing needs for housing, medical care, vocational training that may need to be addressed before treatment for mental health–substance use problems can be successful.

NATIONAL DUAL DIAGNOSIS PROGRAMME

The National Dual Diagnosis Programme was established by the National Institute for Mental Health in response to this national guidance,[6] to improve and develop services for this complex and often excluded group of individuals.

The National Dual Diagnosis Programme adopted a practical approach to supporting regional developments in mental health–substance use, and was interested to clarify what professionals and individuals using services felt was required at the clinical interface to improve services for the individual, family and carers. An informal survey over a number of months with clinicians, families and people who were attending services resulted in a number of generalised themes for development.
➤ Professionals did not feel confident about working with people experiencing mental health–substance use problems.

➤ Professionals and carers did not feel they had the capabilities to effectively support people experiencing mental health–substance use problems.
➤ Carers and families often felt unsupported and felt there were no mechanisms that allowed them to work cooperatively with treatment services.
➤ There were few examples of strategic developments for mental health–substance use problems.
➤ Assertive Outreach and Early Intervention Teams were reporting very high numbers of individuals experiencing mental health–substance use problems.

A commissioned review of former policy recommendations relative to mental health–substance use[9] gave a focus on areas of consistent policy concern (*see* Reference 9 for additional information).

The National Dual Diagnosis Programme felt that there was a 'foundation' stage in implementing the principles of the *Dual Diagnosis Good Practice Guide*,[10] which needed to address the underpinning issues of capabilities, training, strategic development, information and knowledge sharing, and the lack of mental health–substance use service mapping information for in England.

The role of Assertive Outreach Teams in delivering effective services to people experiencing mental health–substance use problems was clearly articulated in a number of policy statements. Indeed, the original team specification described in the Mental Health Policy Implementation Guide[5] indicates that the whole team should have the core skills to assess and manage mental health–substance use problems. This became the starting point for designing a whole-team training package piloted in Assertive Outreach Teams. A number of important issues were highlighted that were relevant not only for the future of assertive outreach mental health–substance use training but for other skills-based continuing professional development courses.[9] These included:

➤ Support and training for trainers to ensure fidelity to materials and quality of delivery.
➤ Time to release the professional for training.
➤ The involvement of other relevant professionals (e.g. substance use professionals and or mental health professionals).
➤ The involvement of the individual in delivery.
➤ Issues around continued supervision and advice in clinical practice in order to translate learning into longer-term changes to how both the professional and the professional team works alongside individuals experiencing mental health–substance use problems.

The National Dual Diagnosis Programme also supports providers and commissioners by developing products that bring together best practice and innovation and address some of the gaps in current service provision, by providing a consistent approach across localities, whilst adapting to local need in line with national policy guidance.

The development of a library resource was one of the early products produced by the programme that brought together information in a CD-ROM format on mental health–substance use policy, research, and good practice, alongside local examples of training and policy programmes that had been developed around the country. This later evolved into a web-based resource, (*see* To learn more) linked to a website that promotes leadership in mental health–substance use through a group of consultant nurses across England, known as the 'Progress' Group

The notion of bringing people together, who were often working in isolation, was another key aim of the National Dual Diagnosis Programme, and a number of regional forums and networks were developed that enabled front-line professionals, the individual experiencing mental health–substance use problems, the family, carers and commissioners, to come together and work through many of the barriers presented to developing local integrated treatment services.

A DVD and handbook (*see* To learn more) was produced that gave the family and carers an opportunity to talk frankly about how their contact with treatment services could be improved, and highlighted the values and approaches that they found most helpful.

NATIONAL SERVICE FRAMEWORK DEVELOPMENT

The autumn assessment of mental health has been an annual event since the National Service Framework was launched in 1999.[16] Its purpose was to provide an in depth assessment of the progress of services towards full implementation of the National Service Framework, and was comprised of four main strands:

1 A self-assessment process on local services carried out by Local Implementation Teams.
2 Finance mapping.
3 Mapping of adult mental health services.
4 A themed review on a key topic.

This review,[17] and the detailed local and national reports[18] that result from it, were designed to help evaluate local progress, on both specific targets, and the development of mental health services. The themed review key topic for the autumn assessment of mental health in 2006–2007 was mental health–substance use.[17]

One of the main aims of this review was to encourage integration between substance use expertise and related training into mental health provision, to provide a standard service plan. The review also wanted to investigate what quantitative and qualitative information was available about services for people of all ages with both mental health and substance use needs. The review encompassed local strategic plans, service delivery, health promotion and the training needs of the professional.

THEMES IDENTIFIED FROM LOCAL IMPLEMENTATION TEAMS

There were five key themes to the information, returned from over 80% of the Local Implementation Teams across England:[17]

1 Definitions and integration of services

Almost all of the Local Implementation Teams reported having a local definition of mental health–substance use in place. However, 40% did not have a mental health–substance use strategy agreed with local stakeholders. With regard to integration between mental health and substance use services, there was evidence of some progress in this vital area. However, local leadership and championing of mental health–substance use was still lacking in many areas.

2 Resourcing and planning

The majority of Local Implementation Teams reported that individuals experiencing mental health–substance use problems were either having a severe or quite severe resource impact on mental health services, with only 2% reporting little impact. Despite this, some basic cornerstones for planning services such as local needs assessment and monitoring had only been achieved in a few areas.

3 Satisfaction and outcomes

There was a poor return rate of satisfaction and outcomes from the individual, with two fifths of Local Implementation Teams reporting evidence of this being collated.

4 Public awareness

There was some good information collated around promotion on the impact of substance use and mental health available for the public and the professional. Examples included newsletters, a quarterly bulletin, and a number of information websites run by local Drug and Alcohol Action Teams (*see* To learn more)

5 Skills and capabilities of staff

Training the workforce, and enhancing mental health–substance use knowledge, skills and capabilities remained one of the key challenges across all services. The themed review[17] reported a mixed picture with regard to mental health–substance use training across the country, with wide variances from one-day ad hoc training right through to master's level courses. There were some positive examples of lead nurses with specific mental health–substance use knowledge and skills in admission units, and cross-fertilisation of capabilities between substance use and mental health services.

KEY RECOMMENDATIONS

> **KEY POINT 4.1**
>
> Mental health–substance use is everyone's responsibility and everyone's business.

There were seven key recommendations from the themed review report[17] that modern, effective provision for people experiencing mental health–substance use problems should benefit:

1 **Leadership:** To drive forward change and improve quality in treatment service provision it is imperative that there is clear designated local leadership for the strategic development of mental health–substance use to involving all key stakeholders. Practice experience suggests that where there is a lead person within a

locality, this keeps mental health–substance use on the agenda, and ensures it remains everyone's responsibility and everyone's business.

2 **Joint strategic needs assessment:** This is a key tool to help raise awareness around mental health–substance use issues locally. Data can help plan and target where service improvement and development is required, from the less intensive end of the spectrum, including those with less severe mental health–substance use difficulties, through to individuals with more severe mental health–substance use problems.

3 **Individual involvement and development of outcomes:** Involvement of the individual experiencing mental health–substance use problems, the family and carers should be at the centre of all work, from initial assessment and engagement process through to being a key voice in strategy development and monitoring the quality of treatment services provided. It was recommended[17] that services recorded effectiveness through the individual(s) defined by the individual outcomes and worked towards a local outcomes framework for mental health–substance use.

4 **Workforce:** The skills and capabilities of the mental health and substance use professional is key to progressing the agenda, alongside service improvement techniques. There have been some tools developed to assist with this process, such as the Dual Diagnosis Capability Framework,[11] and the Ten Essential Shared Capability Module for Dual Diagnosis.[12] Often, when individuals are passed from service to service, it is due to professionals lack of confidence and competence in dealing with mental health–substance use problems. Developing an understanding of the issues, and having a good structure, of personal and professional development within an organisational training framework, is key to developing and improving the skills of the professional.

5 **Strategic development and ownership:** This is key to all the recommendations and should include the development of training needs as part of the overall mental health–substance use strategy development and implementation.

6 **Co-ordination of care:** Due to the complexities and challenges of working with the individual experiencing mental health–substance use problems, robust assessment processes need to be implemented. There should be a holistic approach to care including particular attention to physical, psychological and social needs.

7 **Commissioning for outcomes:** There should be effective recording of user-defined outcomes leading to a locally developed outcomes framework for dual diagnosis.

NEW HORIZONS

The recommendations gave the National Dual Diagnosis Programme a refreshed focus, and it continues to support leadership, education and capable practitioners,[13] and has published strategy guidance.[10] It has held regional events across England to encourage strategy developments based on regional intelligence and local assessment of need.

The new decade, commencing 2010, sees a shift in the direction and principles that govern the direction of national policy for mental health and well-being. 'New

Horizons'[14] focuses on the values and ideologies that strengthen a future care system that is underpinned by the following principles – all have implications for the future of mental health–substance use services in England:

> **Early intervention:** to improve long-term outcomes.
> **Prevention and public mental health:** recognising the need to prevent, and treat mental health problems and promote mental health and well-being.
> **Working with stigma:** a focus on social inclusion and tackling stigma and discrimination wherever they occur.
> **Personalised care:** ensuring that care is based on individuals' needs and wishes, leading to recovery.
> **Multi-agency commissioning/collaboration:** working to achieve a joint approach between local authorities, the National Health Service and others, mirrored by cross-government collaboration.
> **Innovation:** seeking out new and dynamic ways to achieve our objectives based on research and new technologies.
> **Value for money:** delivering cost-effective and innovative services in a period of recession.
> **Strengthening transition:** improving the transition from child and adolescent mental health services to adult services, for those with continuing needs.

New Horizons,[14] sets out an intention across a wide range of agencies moving towards a society where people understand that in order to live life to the full, mental health and well-being is equally as important as physical health. It is a cross-government programme of action aiming to improve mental health and well-being of the population, and improve the quality and accessibility of services for people with poor mental health. New Horizons[14] reminds us that:

> Dual diagnosis is one of the most challenging problems in mental health care and requires collaborative working between a number of different agencies. It is particularly associated with the work of assertive outreach and offender mental health teams, but is sufficiently common for dual diagnosis skills to be essential in all frontline services.

Here, mental health–substance use is identified as one of the key areas for continuation of service improvement across mental health and substance use policy and practice. Although the Department of Health, England, has issued a number of documents that provide guidance on assessment, developing care plans, and delivering care with outcomes in mind, there are still a number of key actions identified within New Horizons[14] including:

> To continue the development of training initiatives to encourage and promote joint working between mental health and substance use services:
>   — National Dual Diagnosis Programme has developed a series of bespoke training materials referenced to the Dual Diagnosis Capabilities Framework 12 and based on the original Assertive Outreach Team training programme – to support Crisis Teams; Early Intervention Teams;

Community Mental Health Teams – and for those working in the criminal justice system.
➤ Training in the care of substance use for mental health professionals:
— National Dual Diagnosis Programme has developed a training pack aimed specifically at acute admission mental health professionals, which will inform developments in improving the acute care pathways for individuals with a mental health–substance use problems.
➤ Priority for mental health–substance use under the Care Programme Approach – the new guidance[15] stipulates the importance of assessing substance use. Having a care plan related to this, and for professionals to be trained to work with people with mental health–substance use problems. Substance use should be considered in all assessments undertaken by mental health services.

CONCLUSION

In taking forward New Horizons[14] principles, policy guidance and the recommendations from the themed review,[17] local areas and strategic health authorities will need to raise the priority of mental health–substance use as a system deliverable. Effective services influence a number of key health and social care issues, in domains, such as physical health, public health, education, employment and accommodation. However, in its own right, mental health–substance use does not feature highly in the operating frameworks in any of these areas, including mental health.

Local leadership is paramount in raising the profile of mental health–substance use, and in developing the local and national evidence base, in terms of clinical and economic arguments. Levers to promote investment in services need to be articulated, argued and won to ensure a future focus for mental health–substance use – and to ensure that people who experience mental health–substance use problems, the family and the carers are treated by recovery-orientated services that are sensitive, humane and effective.

REFERENCES

1 Department of Health. *Mental Health Policy Implementation Guide.* London: Department of Health; 2001. Available at: www.dh.gov.uk/prod_consum_dh/groups/dh_digitalassets/@dh/@en/documents/digitalasset/dh_4058960.pdf (accessed 3 June 2010).
2 Home Office. *Tackling Drugs to Build a Better Britain: the Government's 10-year strategy for tackling drug misuse.* London: HMSO; 1998.
3 Home Office. *Updated Drugs Strategy.* London: HMSO; 2002.
4 National Treatment Agency for Substance Misuse. *Model of Care for the Treatment of Adult Drug Misusers: update 2006.* London: Department of Health and Home Office; 2006. Available at: www.nta.nhs.uk/publications/documents/nta_modelsofcare_update_2006_moc3.pdf (accessed 3 June 2010).
5 Department of Health. *Mental Health Policy Implementation Guide: community mental health teams.* London: Department of Health; 2002. Available at: www.mentalhealthnurse.co.uk/images/DoH%20Guidance/PIG%20CMHT.pdf (accessed 3 June 2010).
6 Department of Health. *Mental Health Practice Implementation Guide: dual diagnosis good*

practice guide. London: Department of Health; 2002. Available at: www.substancemisuserct. co.uk/staff/documents/dh_4060435.pdf (accessed 3 June 2010).

7 Evans K. *Dual Diagnosis: a guide for counsellors and case managers*. New York, NY: Guilford Press; 1990.

8 Watson S, Hawking C. *Dual Diagnosis Good Practice Handbook*. London: Turning Point; 2007.

9 Hughes E, Kipping C. Policy context for dual diagnosis service delivery. *Advances in Dual Diagnosis*. 2008; **1**: 4–8.

10 National Mental Health Development Unit. *Developing a Capable Dual Diagnosis Strategy: a good practice guide*. London: Department of Health and National Mental Health Development Unit; 2009. Available at: www.nmhdu.org.uk/silo/files/developing-a-capable-dual-diagnosis-strategy.pdf (accessed 3 June 2010).

11 Hughes E. *Closing the Gap: a capability framework for working effectively with people with combined mental health and substance use problems (dual diagnosis)*. Lincoln: CCAWI, University of Lincoln and Care Services Improvement Programme; 2007. Available at: www. nmhdu.org.uk/silo/files/capability-framework.pdf (accessed 3 June 2010).

12 Essential Shared Capabilities (ESC) Learning Materials Dual Diagnosis. Available at: www. lincoln.ac.uk/ccawi/ESC.htm (accessed 3 June 2010).

13 Care Services Improvement Partnership. *Dual Diagnosis: developing capable practitioners to improve services and increase positive service user experience*. London: Department of Health and Care Services Improvement Partnership; 2008. Available at: www.dualdiagnosis.co.uk/ uploads/documents/originals/CapablePractitioners.pdf (accessed 3 June 2010).

14 Department of Health. *New Horizons: a shared vision for mental health*. London: Department of Health; 2009. Available at: www.dh.gov.uk/en/Publicationsandstatistics/Publications/ PublicationsPolicyAndGuidance/DH_109705 (accessed 9 August 2010).

15 Department of Health. *Refocusing the Care Programme Approach: policy and positive practice guidance*. London: Department of Health; 2008. All resources available at: www.nmhdu.org. uk/nmhdu/en/our-work/improving-mental-health-care-pathways/dual-diagnosis-care-pathways-programme/dual-diagnosis-key-documents/ (accessed 3 June 2010).

16 Department of Health. *National Service Framework for Mental Health*. London: Department of Health; 1999.

17 Department of Health and Care Services Improvement Partnership. *Mental Health NSF Autumn Assessment 2007 – Dual Diagnosis Themed Review*. London: Department of Health and Care Services Improvement Partnership; 2008.

18 Department of Health and NIMHE. *Dual Diagnosis Themed Review Report 2006/7: SHA Regional Reports*. London: Department of Health and NIMHE; 2009.

TO LEARN MORE

- National Mental Health Development Unit (NMHDU) is the agency charged with supporting the implementation of mental health policy in England by the Department of Health in collaboration with the NHS, local authorities and other major stakeholders. For more information visit www.nmhdu.org.uk
- PROGRESS is made up of a group of consultant nurses and expert practitioners who work in the NHS. Their aim is to improve the support and treatment for individuals who have co-existing mental health and alcohol and drug difficulties. For further information visit www. dualdiagnosis.co.uk
- Web-based resources derived from the CD-ROM library resource, and the carer's DVD and booklet can be viewed and accessed at www.dualdiagnosis.co.uk and at www.nmhdu.org.uk

- Local Drug and Alcohol Teams may run information websites, such as www.tameside.gov.uk/drugandalcohol/team at Tameside. An index of Drug and Alcohol Teams is available at http://drugs.homeoffice.gov.uk/dat/directory/

Severe mental health and substance use: developing integrated services – a UK perspective

Hermine L Graham

INTRODUCTION

In the UK, there is an emergence of substantial central guidance on how to meet the needs of the individual experiencing severe mental health and substance use problems. There is growing research literature seeking to identify effective components of service delivery models and treatments.[1-12] However, the question remains as to what impact these have had on UK service delivery, and the outcomes of mental health–substance use problems.

NATIONAL POLICY AND GUIDANCE

In the UK, 2002, the Department of Health developed a number of good practice guides in an attempt to improve the care of those with mental health problems and to aide implementation of innovations in mental health treatment as part of the National Service Framework.[13] Among these was the *Dual Diagnosis Good Practice Guide*.[14] To those immersed in tackling the issue of mental health–substance use problems at that time, such guidance was applauded and welcomed. This was the first centrally issued guidance offering clear definitions and models of service delivery to the mental health service providers and purchasers. Its core messages were of integrated service delivery models and treating mental health–substance use problems within existing mainstream community mental health services, referred to as 'mainstreaming'. However, how prepared were mainstream services to deliver the recommendations of this guidance?

The policy acknowledged the importance of training professionals within mental health services to facilitate the shift to integrated service delivery. However, a training needs analysis carried out as part of the Dual Diagnosis Information Project[15] revealed that 55% of the sample felt '*inadequately prepared to work with this client group*'.[15] Moreover, respondents reported that poor availability and quality of training, excess workloads and lack of available funds were significant barriers to them accessing the necessary training.

In 2006, mental health–substance use problems were identified as a significant issue related to increased psychiatric hospital admissions, and negatively impacting on treatment during in-patient stays. Hence, guidance was developed to improve assessment and management of mental health–substance use problems on mental health admission and day hospital settings.[16] It identified that 22%–44% of individuals admitted for mental health problems also had co-existing substance use problems. This guidance spoke of the necessity of sufficiently trained professionals so that co-existing substance use is treated as part of the clinical management strategy of a psychiatric admission.[16] Nonetheless, subsequent reviews have continued to highlight the need for improvements in service provision for mental health–substance use problems, not only within community settings but also in inpatient units.[17,18]

In the themed review of *Dual Diagnosis* (2007), Louis Appleby, National Director for Mental Health, reiterated:

> The management of people with dual diagnosis remains an area of concern and one of high priority for mental health policy and within clinical practice. This was highlighted in the National Service Framework for Mental Health – 5 years on document,17 where I restated that dual diagnosis remained one of the biggest challenges for mental health service providers.[18]

This review aimed, for the first time, to assess the extent to which the *Dual Diagnosis Good Practice Guide*[14] had been implemented within services. Eighty per cent (n = 131) of services responded. Although in most services, there were agreed definitions of mental health–substance use problems, and '*evidence of progress towards better integration with mainstream mental health services*', 40% of services had not moved beyond this to have agreed mental health–substance use strategies, and the majority of services did not have local leadership focused on mental health–substance use problems.[18]

The Healthcare Commission review[19] of acute inpatient services found that adequate steps have not been taken to address the treatment of mental health–substance use problems on inpatient units. It stated:

> Despite the high levels of co-morbid mental health and substance misuse problems, only 26% of clinical staff reported having had training from their trust at any time in how to ask service users about their use of alcohol or drugs (including illegal drugs) and only 22% reported having had training in how to handle patients who are drunk or under the influence of drugs.[19]

The conclusions were that commissioners and providers of mental health services should take action to ensure appropriate and safe interventions are provided. It further recommended that more professional training is needed, and to provide specialist services for the individual experiencing mental health problems and who use substances, and that they should focus on '*developing expertise in working with people with a Dual Diagnosis*'.

The poor findings of the reviews of policy guidance for mental health–substance use problems in both community and inpatient settings perhaps, to some extent, reflect the challenges of developing integrated service provision within ever evolving, pressured mental health services with a number of areas identified as priorities that need to be addressed simultaneously. Hence, the question remains for consideration: what factors positively influence the development and implementation of a coordinated service response for those experiencing mental health–substance use problems?

INTERNATIONAL CONTEXT AND DEVELOPMENTS

In a number of countries (e.g. USA, New Zealand, Australia) there have been attempts to develop coordinated service responses to the issue of mental health–substance use. One New Hampshire, USA, study reviewed the development and evolution of mental health–substance use approaches since the 1980s, and a number of controlled research studies carried out during the 1990s.[3,4] These researchers and service developers have gone a long way toward identifying what continues to be described as the common '*critical components*' of an integrated treatment approach (i.e. staged interventions, assertive outreach, motivational interventions, counselling, social support interventions, long-term perspective, comprehensiveness, cultural sensitivity and competence). This study identified a number of barriers to implementation. Similar to the position in the UK, it described poor levels of implementation, despite favourable research evidence and integrated treatment being viewed positively and widely advocated. In the USA, the key barriers to the implementation of integrated treatment for mental health–substance use problems included:

➤ separately commissioned, funded and delivered mental health and substance use services
➤ a lack of a clear local service delivery model
➤ professionals being insufficiently trained and familiar with working with both substance use and mental health, and a lack of awareness of the impact of substance use on the individual and the family.

It is important to note that poor implementation of interventions within mental health services is not unique to mental health–substance use. Another study,[20] suggests that despite interventions being evidence based and adopted within policy-frameworks, the reasons influencing poor implementation are numerous, but: '*In part, the roots of this treatment quality crisis lie in the unsystematic evolution of treatments for SMI during the past 40 years.*'[20]

COMBINED PSYCHOSIS AND SUBSTANCE USE (COMPASS) PROGRAMME, BIRMINGHAM, UK

In Birmingham, UK, we came against some of the barriers to the development and implementation of innovative mental health practice and sought to tackle these challenges.[21] The service setting was Northern Birmingham Mental Health Trust (NBMHT), a provider of mental health and substance use services to an urban catchment population of approximately 570 000. This inner-city area was classified as having high social deprivation, ranked fifth in the country.[23] The 1991 National Census unemployment rates between different localities in the region ranged from 5%–28%. The area was also a blend of cultural/racial groups, and 'minority populations' (Asian, from the Indian sub-continent and Black, typically African-Caribbean), ranged from 3%–69% in the different localities of the region.[24]

As part of the shift within the UK to deliver community-based treatment services for people who experience severe mental health problems,[25] Northern Birmingham Mental Health had evolved into a provider of functionalised Community Mental Health Teams, derived from community-based treatment models. The teams included:
> locality-based Primary Care Mental Health Liaison Teams
> Home Treatment Teams (*see* refs. 26–7)
> Rehabilitation and Recovery Teams
> Assertive Outreach Teams (*see* Refs. 25–30). Substance use service provision were geographically based community drug teams, inpatient services, a community alcohol team and a specialist crack-cocaine service. These services were based on a harm-reduction philosophy rather than abstinence.[31,32]

In a survey of the prevalence of substance use problems among those with severe mental health problems across Northern Birmingham's mental health and substance use services, of 3079 individuals sampled, 1369 were identified as having a severe mental health diagnosis (defined as psychotic disorders, bipolar disorders and major depressive disorders), classified according to ICD-10 criteria. Based on professional reports, 24% of individuals (324/1369) had used alcohol and/or drugs problematically in the past year.[33] Similar to other services across the UK,[34,35] it was evident that, the needs of those with mental health–substance use problems were not being met by existing separate service provision.[36] A number of factors appeared to contribute to this:

1 Provision of treatment for substance use was provided in parallel to mental health treatment. Thus, substance use and mental health services, although provided by the same organisation, were structurally and geographically separate. Those with mental health–substance use problems did not fit neatly into these well-defined services, and often fell somewhere between the two. Additionally, liaison between the two types of services was variable, depending on who dealt with an enquiry or referral.

2 The treatment and engagement philosophies of the two types of services differed significantly. Mental health services tended to adopt a more assertive approach to engaging the individual in treatment, whether the individual felt they had mental health problems or not. In contrast, substance use services in the UK have typically required motivation for change as a prerequisite for treatment to be offered.

3 The focus of the two types of services, in terms of assessment and treatment, was on either mental health or substance use.

4 Based on a training needs survey of 136 professionals across community-based mental health and substance use services, each service tended to focus on their area of expertise, and the professional although willing to work with mental

health–substance use problems, generally lacked the confidence, skills and basic knowledge to do so.[37]

The need to provide an adequate service response for individuals with mental health–substance use problems was the setting for a fundamental shift in service provision. In an attempt to address this gap the Combined Psychosis and Substance Use (COMPASS) Programme was a new initiative targeted at the local level of service delivery that aimed at integrating existing service provision and building the capabilities of the professional. The necessary extra resources to kick-start developments were made available through an application for centrally allocated resources. The resulting service model and treatment approach, highlighted as a model of good practice within the *Dual Diagnosis Good Practice Guide*[14] has been developed, implemented and evaluated.[38,39] A number of lessons have been learned from this process. It is from this experience, and the available literature and research, that some of the key issues necessary for the development and implementation of services for mental health–substance use problems will be considered.

Engagement of key stakeholders
One study[3,4] highlighted separately commissioned, funded and delivered mental health and substance use services as one of the key barriers to implementation. It can be suggested that a number of factors facilitated joint commissioning, ownership and support for the implementation of an integrated approach to mental health–substance use within Northern Birmingham. Key stakeholders were engaged in this process of shifting the focus of mainstream mental health services toward including mental health–substance use problems and integrating it within its core business. A multi-agency steering group (commissioners, strategic health authority lead, social care lead, probation, etc.), and a number of steering groups within NBMHT (local managers and service directors; research and development group), were put in place to direct and facilitate the development and implementation of this initiative. Team managers were involved from the pilot and developmental stages. The training and intervention developed was based on the outcomes of the local training and need assessment carried out across the organisation.[40]

Locally relevant services
The literature highlights that although there are a number of effective evidence-based interventions in mental health, few of them are implemented in routine practice.[20,41] The suggestion is that service innovations and developments are more likely to occur, and be maintained, if they are perceived as being locally relevant and can be implemented easily within existing practice. A lack of a clear local service delivery model was identified as a barrier to implementation.[3,4] The paucity of UK prevalence and treatment evaluation during the late 1990s, meant that there was insufficient information on a national and local level to guide the service developments in Northern Birmingham. However, visits to leading mental health–substance use services in the USA emphasised that although a lot could be learned from these services and treatment approaches, these models could not be wholly imported and implemented in the UK due to non-local relevance. There

are significant differences in the contextual factors that guide service provision in the two countries.[22,36]

Strategic planning

In an attempt to ensure the approach developed in Northern Birmingham was locally relevant, a strategic plan directed the intervention. One study,[20] suggests that a significant barrier to the implementation of evidenced-based interventions within the mental health field has been the *'unsystematic evolution of practice'*. Perhaps this suggests that the lack of a clear, purposeful and strategic approach to innovation has hindered implementation. The strategic plan that directed the development of the COMPASS Programme seemed to 'naturally' emerge from the steering groups and the findings of the research that was carried out to identify local needs in the context of the growing body of research evidence available at that time.

The first stage of the strategic plan involved consulting with key stakeholders. It incorporated a first stage of mapping local need, which included assessments of prevalence,[33] staff training and support needs.[40] This survey identified the number of people with mental health–substance use problems and pointed to where the majority of these individuals were located, and the greatest need lay. The training needs assessment of 136 community-based professionals revealed that they had frequent contact with these individuals, were interested in working with the individual, and saw it as part of their professional role. However, the professionals felt they needed more information and training to improve their knowledge and skills to enable confident practice alongside the individual.[40]

The information gathered during the mapping stage provided a clear, purposeful, and strategic approach to the innovation of services for mental health–substance use problems within the Trust. However, it must be emphasised that although the overall strategic plan was endorsed at the multi-agency and Trust board level, the details at the operational level of what the remit of the integrated service provision would be, i.e. a mental health–substance use team that would essentially be a third service with a caseload or a specialist team that trained and supported existing services. In addition, where it would be located (i.e. mental health or substance use services) evoked considerable debate and tension.[36] The latter continues to be a bone of contention and perhaps both issues are significant sticking points in many other National Health Service (NHS) Trusts. This contributed to the finding of the Themed Review of Dual Diagnosis that 40% of services had not moved beyond agreed definitions to have agreed mental health–substance use strategies.[18]

Model of service delivery

Based on the results of the assessment of local need, a review of the evidence base and developments elsewhere, an 'integrated shared care' model was developed that sought to complement the existing service provision. The model aimed to achieve integration of treatment,[3,42] not only at the professional level but also at service level. The key principle underlying this integration was that both mental health and substance use needs are addressed at the same time by *'mainstream mental health services'*.[14] The idea was that in the main this would be done by the mental health professionals but in some cases it could be achieved via shared-care/liaison between mental health and substance use services. If there is integration at the service level then this ensures that access to specialist substance use is available. In addition, integration at the service level means that there are agreed protocols for closer and/ or joint working between mental health and substance use services.

The service delivery model chosen was one where the COMPASS Programme team became a specialist intra- and inter-disciplinary team to 'champion' the integrated approach at a local and strategic level. It served to provide training, support and consultancy to existing professionals and build a bridge between substance use and mental health services in a 'hub and spoke' fashion. The model was opposed to creating an additional specialist third service that took on a mental health–substance use caseload due to the pitfalls inherent within such an approach.[13,36] It can be suggested that integrated treatment was achieved, to its greatest extent, in the Assertive Outreach Teams. This is due to the large proportion of mental health–substance use problems located within these teams, and the integrated service model fitting with the philosophy of the Programme in Assertive Community Treatment model.[28–30]

WHERE TO TARGET RESOURCES

It was decided to initially focus on, and target, resources at mental health services and the individual using the service experiencing severe mental health problems – rather than the individual with more common mental health problems, or primarily personality-related difficulties. The rationale for this was driven by where individuals were located, the gap in service provision and ability to access necessary services. Individuals with more common mental health problems are generally better able to negotiate their way between mental health and substance use services to access appropriate help. In contrast, the individual experiencing severe mental health problems is less able to do this and often 'falls between the gap'.[43,44] Moreover, prevalence rates were higher,[45] and outcomes poorer.[46–48]

Assertive Outreach Teams

Two key issues led to the deployment of the bulk of the resources to mental health services and to Assertive Outreach Teams:

1 The results of the survey of prevalence identified that 83% of people experiencing mental health–substance use problems were located within mental health teams. Analysis revealed that a significantly greater number of individuals experiencing severe mental health problems, who were also using substances, were located in Assertive Outreach Teams. The individuals represented a range of 26%–45% of Assertive Outreach Teams' caseloads.[49]

2 There was a need for the individual experiencing severe mental health problems to remain engaged, and managed, within Assertive Outreach Teams, in line with the model, on which, this is based,[28] and effective demonstration studies using a similar approach to that of the USA.[1,50]

Acute inpatient services and Primary Care Mental Health Teams

The results of the assessment of prevalence across mental health and substance use services indicated that, although mental health teams (teams other than Assertive Outreach), and substance use services did not have the highest proportion of individuals experiencing severe mental health and substance use problems, a number of individual experiencing mental health–substance use problems were still present in these services.[33] It was clear from consultations with these services, and the assessment of need, that they did not require the intensive input of Assertive Outreach Teams. However, difficulties were experienced when accessing specialist services. They felt they lacked particular skills and knowledge to carry out specialist assessment, and offer brief motivational-based interventions.[40] Consequently, a different approach was taken to improve the capabilities of these services to respond to mental health–substance use problems. The focus was on providing training in brief motivational interventions, improving access to specialist assessment and services for acute inpatient facilities, and non-assertive outreach community mental health teams and substance use services.[51]

Training

In the UK, improving the skills and expertise of the professional to work in an integrated manner, and address problematic substance use in the individual who experiences mental health–substance use problems, has been flagged as a major objective to improve outcomes in both community and inpatient mental health services.[14,16–19] One study,[3,4] highlight insufficiently trained professionals, unfamiliar with working with both substance use and mental health, and lacking awareness of the impact of substance use on the individual and family, as a barrier to integration.[3,4]

The main training needs, for mental health professionals, identified from training needs analyses in the UK are:

➤ information about substances and mental health–substance use problems, the skills to work with the individual and information on how to access specialist services[40]
➤ psychological interventions (e.g. motivational interviewing, cognitive behavioural therapy)
➤ issues of diagnosis/assessment
➤ treatment/management issues.[15]

The Dual Diagnosis in Mental Health Inpatient and Day Hospital Settings policy recommended that professionals in inpatient settings be trained to use '*simple motivational interventions*' as an attempt to '*improve motivation and encourage behaviour change, to prevent relapse and minimise harm*'.[16] The '*core competencies*' identified in the *Dual Diagnosis Good Practice Guide*,[14] (2002) and the Dual Diagnosis Capability Framework[52] to improve the ability of professionals to work with mental health–substance use problems are:

➤ perceiving mental health–substance use problems as part of the core role
➤ attitudes to working with mental health–substance use problems
➤ engagement skills

➤ health promotion
➤ assessment
➤ delivering evidence-based interventions (e.g. motivational interventions, relapse prevention and early signs monitoring)
➤ ability to access specialist services.

A number of training models have been described and the difficulties inherent in applying training.[53] The training approach was tailored to the needs of the different types of services.[22,38,51,54] The training specifically developed for Assertive Outreach Teams involved intensive training of the whole team in an attempt to achieve integrated treatment team status. The whole team was trained at the same time, over six half-days; to use Cognitive-behavioural Integrated Treatment (C-BIT).[55] Teams were provided with a manual of the approach and trained to use the intervention. In addition, to achieve the delivery of integrated treatment, teams were provided with a 'change facilitator' (a member of the specialist COMPASS Programme) who worked alongside teams on a weekly basis to continue to train professionals in the Assertive Outreach Teams insitu (and through modelling the skills embodied in the C-BIT approach), and provide supervision. In some instances, this 'product champion' worked jointly on specific cases, on a long-term basis. The aim was to improve the capabilities and capacity of professionals with Assertive Outreach Teams to deliver an integrated treatment (i.e. C-BIT), and to raise the profile of substance use in the team.

The results of the evaluation of the intervention suggests that existing Assertive Outreach Teams experience significant improvements in self-reported confidence and skills relevant to working with mental health–substance use problems, following training, and that these gains are maintained over time. These results were replicated in two teams trained after an 18-month delay.[54,56] This study suggests that training mental health professionals (trained and untrained) to use an integrated treatment approach is well received and produces lasting changes in confidence and skills.

Our experience suggests that to significantly impact, long term, on the confidence and skills of professionals working within existing Assertive Outreach Teams, training needs to include a number of factors:

1 Adopting a 'team approach' to the delivery of training

A number of studies that focus on the issue of training within mental health settings suggest that providing the professional with training does not necessary result in using or transferring the newly acquired skills into the clinical setting.[57–59] To facilitate a shift in the treatment philosophy of an existing team to embrace the concept of integrated treatment all professionals within the team, need to be trained, and preferably at the same time. It has been suggested that training a single team member does not change the treatment offered by the rest of the team. The importance of training the whole team, as a unit, is that it promotes a paradigm shift within the whole team at the same time.[58] This training method offers all professionals (trained and untrained) within the team an opportunity to be exposed, at the same time, to the issues they feel they may encounter in implementation. The team is then able to work through these issues and resolve them as a team.

2 *Providing ongoing in situ training, co-working, modelling and supervision*

Ongoing in situ training/modelling, co-working and supervision were an inbuilt part of the training package. Once professionals' were trained they were allocated a member of the COMPASS Programme team who would work alongside, two days per week, on a long-term basis. This person served as a 'product champion' who modelled the approach within the team setting, developed integrated treatment/care plans and co-worked with the individual alongside the team and key workers.[38,42,54,61] In addition, this role provided specialist team-supervision sessions. The aim of these sessions was to facilitate the process whereby the professional team is able, using the new treatment approach, to think through a particular scenario, in light of his/her case formulation, and refine treatment plans.[62] Evidence from training in psychosocial interventions for substance use as part of the United Kingdom Alcohol Treatment Trial,[35] demonstrates the importance of incorporating supervision into training packages. They found that supervision was pivotal in the maintenance of competence in delivering the intervention post training.[63]

3 *Address attitudes/perceptions*

A major hurdle in implementing an integrated treatment approach are the attitudes and perceptions of the professional.[3,4,13,52,64,65] Some mental health professionals continue to perceive mental health–substance use problems as of the individual's own volition – intractable – and feel pessimistic about the effectiveness of any treatment. In addition, some believe that the treatment of substance use is out of their remit and area of expertise.[66] Merely offering skills-based training would not necessarily improve motivation to engage with the individual experiencing mental health–substance use problems unless underlying attitudes are addressed.

Qualitative interviews exploring the attitudes of mental health professionals to cannabis and crack-cocaine use revealed that there are different attitudes to different substances and this may influence what, if any, interventions are offered.[64,65] Professionals adjusted their approach to intervening with cannabis users dependent on the impact they felt it was having on the individual, whether they felt any intervention would jeopardise the therapeutic relationship, and their own personal/professional view.[65] Hence effective training programmes need to facilitate a shift in professional attitudes toward working with substance use and psychosis. Key strategies that serve to do so during training are psychoeducation and building empathy. Psychoeducation during the training of the Assertive Outreach Teams included information about prevalence, social, cognitive and motivational obstacles to change, awareness of the relapsing nature of substance use problems via the stages of change model (*see* Book 4, Chapter 6).[67]

Empathy is a means through which attitudes can be addressed. It encourages engagement and the building of shared understandings, collaborative relationships, and therapeutic alliances. It has been suggested that empathy is a key factor in establishing a positive therapeutic relationship and working alliance.[68] However, professionals may find it harder to develop empathy when faced with 'symptoms' they perceive as being outside the scope of their own experience and expertise.[68] Therefore, training professionals to elicit the individual's cognitions, and developing individualised case formulations, can serve to enhance empathy in therapeutic relationships. Encouraging the Assertive Outreach Teams to use scenarios from their caseloads as examples when carrying out training exercises helped to facilitate this process. These included:

➤ eliciting and understanding the individual's substance-related beliefs and reasons for continued substance use
➤ the development of individualised case formulations
➤ encouraging the adoption of a long-term, optimistic, and stage-wise approach to the identification of individual treatment needs
➤ the development of treatment plans and goals.

4 *User-friendly approach*

For a new treatment approach to be adopted, it needs to be perceived as flexible, user friendly and being compatible, or able to be, incorporated into existing approaches and working routine.[57,69] The integrated approach had been piloted within Assertive Outreach Team settings, and the illustrative case material and style of the treatment approach as documented in the treatment manual that accompanied the training[55] strongly reflected this.

5 *Team ownership and support for implementation*

Training has a greater chance of being transferred, and the behaviour of professionals changed if the training programme has some benefits and rewards and if the professional:

➤ feels involved in the development
➤ takes ownership for implementation
➤ feels that he/she will have time to implement the new skills
➤ receive support from managers
➤ perceives that the individual will benefit.[58,70]

Teams and professionals were engaged as key stakeholders during the development process, and reported that they felt they were getting something out of being involved in the training personally (i.e. skills and training which was university-accredited as a short course), and clinically (i.e. they would receive a specialist professional to work alongside them, with the individual, two days per week, and they had involvement in the innovation).[38]

Sustainability

A number of important lessons were learned during the process of developing and implementing services for mental health–substance use problems in Northern Birmingham. However, the long-term nature of mental health–substance use suggests that attention also needs to be paid to the sustainability of innovations in integrated service provision within ever evolving and pressured mental health services. Some of the factors that appear to influence long-term adoption of demonstration projects include:

➤ professional training
➤ financial commitments/resources

➤ shifting NHS/commissioning priorities
➤ old debates resurfacing about the 'best model' service delivery.

Training programmes need to include:
➤ booster training for existing professionals
➤ training for new professionals.

The nature and frequency of supervision sessions may change over time to reflect the needs of the team and people using the service. Essentially, it is important to try to incorporate team supervision sessions into the Assertive Outreach Teams' routine meeting schedule. We found that the role of the specialist changed over time as the Assertive Outreach Team has adopted the integrated style of working and became more confident. The intensity of and type of support needed changed. After 18 months, the role became more consultancy focused. The professional primarily sought support for individuals with complex needs or who were using substances associated with more social chaos (e.g. crack-cocaine). We noted that the integrated approach was easier to implement in teams who fully utilise the Program for Assertive Community Treatment model (PACT)/Assertive Community Treatment model and team approach, and are sufficiently staffed and resourced.

CONCLUSION

In an evolving National Health Service climate with a substantial number of competing priorities and limited availability of resources, it is essential that organisations prioritise mental health–substance use as a key area for development if any changes are too been seen in the front-line services delivered. Local Champions need to be identified and supported to spearhead the necessary and long overdue developments and improvements in the services received by those who experience severe mental health and substance use problems.

REFERENCES

1 Jerrell JM, Ridgely MS. Evaluating changes in symptoms and functioning of dually diagnosed clients in specialized treatment. *Psychiatr Serv.* 1995; **46**: 233–8.
2 Jerrell JM, Ridgely MS. Impact of robustness of program implementation on outcomes of clients in dual diagnosis programs. *Psychiatr Serv.* 1999; **50**: 109–12.
3 Drake RE, Essock SM, Shaner A, *et al.* Implementing dual diagnosis services for clients with severe mental illness. *Psychiatr Serv.* 2001; **52**: 469–76.
4 Drake RE, Essock SM, Shaner A, *et al.* Implementing dual diagnosis services for clients with severe mental illness. *FOCUS: Journal of Lifelong Learning in Psychiatry.* 2004; **2**(1): 102–10.
5 Barrowclough C, Haddock G, Tarrier N, *et al.* Randomized controlled trial of motivational interviewing, cognitive behavior therapy, and family intervention for patients with comorbid schizophrenia and substance use disorders. *Am J Psychiatry.* 2001; **158**: 1706–13.
6 Haddock G, Barrowclough C, Tarrier N, *et al.* (2003). Cognitive-behavioural therapy and motivational intervention for schizophrenia and substance misuse: 18-month outcomes of a randomized control trial. *Br J Psychiatry.* 2003; **183**; 566–76.

7 Kavanagh D, Young R, White A, *et al.* A brief intervention for substance abuse in early psychosis. *Drug Alcohol Rev.* 2004; **23**: 151–5.

8 Baker A, Bucci S, Lewin TJ, *et al.* Cognitive-behavioural therapy for substance use disorders in people with psychotic disorders: randomised controlled trial. *Br J Psychiatry.* 2006; **188**: 439–48.

9 Edwards J, Elkins K, Hinton M, *et al.* Randomized controlled trial of a cannabis-focused intervention for young people with first-episode psychosis. *Acta Psychiatr Scand.* 2006; **114**: 109–17

10 Baker A, Velleman R, editors. *Clinical Handbook of Co-existing Mental Health and Drug and Alcohol Problems.* London: Routledge; 2007.

11 Cleary M, Hunt GE, Matheson SL, *et al.* Psychosocial interventions for people with both severe mental illness and substance misuse (Review). *The Cochrane Library.* 2008; 4. John Wiley & Sons.

12 Horsfall J, Cleary M, Hunt GE, *et al.* Psychosocial treatments for people with co-occurring severe mental illnesses and substance use disorders (dual diagnosis): a review of empirical evidence. *Harv Rev Psychiatry.* 2009; **18**: 24–34.

13 Department of Health. *The Mental Health Policy Implementation Guide.* 2002. Available at: www.dh.gov.uk/dr_consum_dh/groups/dh_digitalassets/@dh/@en/documents/digital asset/dh_4058960.pdf (accessed 4 June 2010).

14 Department of Health. *Mental Health Policy Implementation Guide: dual diagnosis good practice guide.* London: Department of Health; 2002. Available at: www.dh.gov.uk/dr_ consum_dh/groups/dh_digitalassets/@dh/@en/documents/digitalasset/dh_4060435.pdf (accessed 4 June 2010).

15 Royal College of Psychiatrists. In: Banerjee S, Clancy C, Crome I, editors. *Co-existing problems of mental disorder and substance misuse (dual diagnosis) – An Information Manual.* London: The Royal College of Psychiatrists' Research Unit; 2002.

16 Department of Health. *Dual Diagnosis in mental health inpatient and day hospital settings policy.* Department of Health; 2006. Available at: www.dh.gov.uk/dr_consum_dh/groups/ dh_digitalassets/@dh/@en/documents/digitalasset/dh_062652.pdf (accessed 4 June 2010).

17 Department of Health. *National Service Framework for Mental Health: five years on.* London: Department of Health; 2004.

18 Department of Health / Care Services Improvement Partnership (2007). *Themed Review Report 07: dual diagnosis.* Leeds: Department of Health / Care Services Improvement Partnership.

19 Healthcare Commission. *The Pathway to Recovery: a review of NHS acute inpatient mental health services.* London: Healthcare Commissions; 2008. Available at: www.cqc.org.uk/_ db/_documents/The_pathway_to_recovery_200807251020.pdf (accessed 4 June 2010).

20 Gold PB, Glynn SM, Mueser KT. Challenges to implementing and sustaining comprehensive mental health service programs. *Eval Health Prof.* 2006; **29**: 195–218.

21 Copello A, Graham H, Birchwood M. Evaluating substance misuse interventions in psychosis: The limitations of the RCT with 'patient' as the unit of analysis. Editorial. *J Ment Health.* 2001; **10**: 585–7.

22 Graham HL, Copello A, Birchwood M, *et al.* Co-existing severe mental health and substance use problems: developing integrated services in the UK. *Psychiatr Bull.* 2003; **27**: 183–6.

23 Department of the Environment, Transport and the Regions. *1998 Index of Local Deprivation.* London: Department for Communities and Local Government; 1998. Available at: www. communities.gov.uk/documents/citiesandregions/pdf/155808.pdf (accessed 4 June 2010).

24 1991 UK Census. London: Office for National Statistics; 1991.

25 Department of Health. *National Service Framework for Mental Health: modern standards and service models;* 1999. Available at: www.dh.gov.uk/dr_consum_dh/groups/dh_digital assets/@dh/@en/documents/digitalasset/dh_4077209.pdf (accessed 4 June 2010).

26 Hoult J, Reynolds I. Schizophrenia: a comparative trial of community oriented and hospital oriented psychiatric care. *Acta Psychiatrica Scandinavia.* 1984; **69**: 359–72.

27 Dean C, Gadd EM. Home treatment for acute psychiatric illness. *Br Med J.* 1990; **301**: 1021–3.

28 Stein LI, Test MA. Alternative to mental hospital treatment. *Arch Gen Psychiatry.* 1980; **37**: 392–7.

29 Mcgrew JH, Bond GR. Critical ingredients of assertive community treatment: judgment of the experts. *Assertive Community Treatment* 1995; **22**: 113–25.

30 Drake RE, Burns BJ. Special section on assertive community treatment: an introduction. *Psychiatr Serv.* 1995; **46**: 667–8.

31 Marlatt GA. Basic principles and strategies of harm reduction. In: Marlatt GA, editor. *Harm Reduction: pragmatic strategies for managing high-risk behaviours.* New York, NY: Guilford Publications; 1998.

32 Wilks J. Drug treatment and prescribing practice: what can be learned from the past? In: Bennett G, editor. *Treating Drug Abusers.* London: Routledge; 1989.

33 Graham HL, Maslin J, Copello A, *et al.* Drug and alcohol problems amongst individuals with severe mental health problems in an inner city area of the UK. *Soc Psychiatry Psychiatr Epidemiol.* 2001; **36**: 448–55.

34 Menezes PO, Johnson S, Thornicroft G, *et al.* Drug and alcohol problems amongst individuals with severe mental illness in south London. *Br J Psychiatry.* 1996; **168**: 612–19.

35 Virgo N, Bennett G, Bennett L, Higgins D, Thomas P. (1998). The prevalence of co-occurring severe mental illness and problematic substance misuse (dual diagnosis) in the patients of mental health and addiction services in East Dorset. Poster presented at Addictions '98 conference, Newcastle-upon-Tyne, 25–27 September, 1998.

36 Johnson S. Dual diagnosis of severe mental illness and substance misuse: a case for specialist services? *Br J Psychiatry.* 1997; **171**: 205–8.

37 Maslin J, Graham HL, Cawley M, *et al.* Combined severe mental health and substance use problems: what are the training and support needs of staff working with this client group? *J Ment Health.* 2001; **10**: 131–40.

38 Graham HL. Implementing integrated treatment for co-existing substance use and severe mental health problems in Assertive Outreach Teams: training issues. *Drug Alcohol Rev.* 2004; **23**: 463–70.

39 Graham HL, Copello A, Birchwood M, *et al.* A preliminary evaluation of integrated treatment for co-existing substance use and severe mental health problems: impact on teams and service users. *J Ment Health.* 2006; **15**: 577–91.

40 Maslin J, Graham HL, Cawley M, *et al.* Combined severe mental health and substance use problems: What are the training and support needs of staff working with this client group? *J Ment Health.* 2001; **10**: 131–40.

41 Drake RE, Goldman HH, Leff HS, *et al.* Implementing evidence-based practices in routine mental health service settings. *Psychiatr Serv.* 2001; **52**: 179–82.

42 Mueser KT, Drake RE, Noordsy DL. Integrated mental health and substance abuse treatment for severe psychiatric disorders. *Journal of Psychiatric Practice.* 1998; **4**: 129–39.

43 Franey C, Thom B. The effectiveness of alcohol interventions. In *The Centre for Research on*

Drugs and Health Behaviour, Executive Summary. London: Centre for Research on Drugs and Health Behaviour; **38**: 1995.

44 Rorstad P, Checinski K. Dual diagnosis: facing the challenge. In: Mcgeachy O, Ward M, editors. *Dual diagnosis: meeting the challenge.* London: Wynn Howard; 1996.

45 Regier DA, Farmer ME, Rae DS, *et al.* Comorbidity of mental disorders with alcohol and other drug abuse: results from the Epidemiologic Catchment Area (ECA) study. *J Am Med Assoc.* 1990; **264**: 2511–18.

46 Donald M, Downer J, Kavanagh D. Integrated versus non-integrated management and care for clients with co-occurring mental health and substance use disorders: a qualitative systematic review of randomised controlled trials. *Soc Sci Med.* 2005; **60**: 1371–83.

47 Green AI, Drake RE, Brunette MF, *et al.* Schizophrenia and co-occurring substance use disorder. *Am J Psychiatry.* 2007; **164**: 402–8.

48 Hunt GE, Bergen J, Bashir M. Medication compliance and co-morbid substance abuse in schizophrenia: community survival 4 years after relapse. *Schizophr Res.* 2002; **54**: 253–64.

49 Graham HL. Project update: the combined psychosis and substance use (COMPASS) Programme. *Acquire, Alcohol Concern.* 2002; **33**.

50 Mercer MT, Mueser K, Drake RE. Organizational guidelines for dual disorders programs, *Psychiatr Q.* 1998; **69**: 145–68.

51 Graham HL, Tobin D, Godfrey E. A consultation-liaison service model offering a brief integrated motivational enhancement intervention. In: Baker A, Velleman R, editors. *Clinical Handbook of Co-existing Mental Health and Drug and Alcohol Problems.* Hove: Routledge and New York: Routledge; 2007.

52 Hughes, L. *Closing the Gap: a capability framework for working effectively with people with people with combined mental health and substance use problems (dual diagnosis).* London: Department of Health / Care Services Improvement Partnership; 2006.

53 Crome I, Bloor R. Training in co-existing mental health and drug and alcohol problems: High priority in policy requires resources. In: Baker A, Velleman R, editors. *Clinical Handbook of Co-existing Mental Health and Drug and Alcohol Problems.* Hove: Routledge; 2007. pp. 351–70.

54 Graham HL, Copello A, Birchwood M, *et al.* A preliminary evaluation of integrated treatment for co-existing substance use and severe mental health problems: impact on teams and service users. *J Ment Health.* 2006; **15**: 577–91.

55 Graham HL, Copello A, Birchwood MJ, *et al. Cognitive-behavioural Integrated Treatment (C-BIT): a treatment manual for substance misuse in people with severe mental health problems.* Chichester: John Wiley & Sons; 2004.

56 Graham HL. Implementing integrated treatment for co-existing substance use and severe mental health problems in Assertive Outreach Teams: training issues. *Drug Alcohol Rev.* 2004; **23**: 463–70.

57 Kavanagh DJ. Issues in multidisciplinary training of cognitive-behavioural interventions. *Behav Change.* 1994; **11**: 38–44.

58 Corrigan PW, McCracken SG. *Interactive Staff Training: rehabilitation teams that work.* New York: Plenum Press; 1997.

59 Milne D, Gorenski O, Westerman C, *et al.* What does it take to transfer training? *Psychiatr Rehabil Skills.* 2000; **4**: 259–81.

60 Miller WR, Mount KA. (2001). A small study of training in motivational interviewing: Does one workshop change clinician and client behaviour? *Behav Cogn Psychother.* **29**: 457–71.

61 Copello A, Tobin D. Clinical team supervision for practitioners treating co-existing mental

health and drug and alcohol problems. In: Baker A, Velleman R, editors. *Clinical Handbook of Co-existing Mental Health and Drug and Alcohol Problems.* Hove: Routledge; 2007.

62 Tober G, Godfrey C, Parrott S, *et al.* Setting standards for training and competence: the UK alcohol treatment trial. *Alcohol Alcohol.* 2005; **40**: 413–18.

63 Clutterbuck R, Tobin D, Orford J, *et al.* Exploring the attitudes of staff working within mental health settings toward clients who use cannabis. *Drugs: Educ, Prev Polic.* 2009; **16**: 311–27.

65 Clutterbuck R, Tobin D, Orford J, *et al.* Staff attitudes towards cocaine/crack-cocaine use amongst individuals with severe mental health problems in an inner city area of the UK. *Ment Health and Subst Use.* 2008; **1**: 205–15.

66 Derricott J, Mckeown M. Dual diagnosis: future directions in training. *Psychiatr Care.* 1996; **3**: 34–7.

67 Prochaska JO, DiClemente CC, Norcross JC. In search of how people change: applications to addictive behaviours. *Am Psychol.* 1992; **47**: 1102–14.

68 McLeod H, Deane FP, Hogbin B. Changing staff attitudes and empathy for working with people with psychosis. *Behav Cogn Psychother.* 2002; **30**: 459–70.

69 Milne D, Woodward K, Hanner S. An illustration of delivering evidence-based practice through staff training: multi-dimensional process, outcome and organisational evaluation. *Behav Cogn Psychother.* 2003; **31**: 85–98.

70 Milne D, Gorenski O, Westerman C, Leck, *et al.* What does it take to transfer training? *Psychiatr Rehabil Skills.* 2000; **4**: 259–81.

An Australian rural service system's journey towards systemic mental health–substance use capability

Gary J Croton

PRE-READING EXERCISE 6.1

Time: 60–90 minutes
- Download from the 'Tools' section of www.dualdiagnosis.org.au an 'agency dual diagnosis capability checklist'.[1,2] (either Victorian or non-Victorian versions)
- Complete for your agency including the development of a draft plan for further developing your agency's level of mental health–substance use capability.

Be mindful that completing the checklist would normally be a whole team activity.

INTRODUCTION
Systemic mental health–substance use capability defined
Systemic mental health–substance use capability may be defined as the capacity of a healthcare system to recognise and effectively respond to persons experiencing mental health–substance use problems. Since 1998, the mental health and drug treatment arms of the Eastern Hume healthcare system have allocated resources to developing systemic mental health–substance use capability. This chapter outlines the context of this development process, provides an Eastern Hume 'progress report' and describes strategies found successful in the pursuit of systemic mental health–substance use capability.

DEMOGRAPHICS, SERVICES AND RURAL CHALLENGE
Demographics
The Eastern Hume region lies in the northeast of Victoria, Australia; it covers 23 000 square km and has a population of 120 000. The region is substantially rural with two main urban centres, Wangaratta and Wodonga, and a number of smaller towns.

Over the last decade, Eastern Hume has experienced significant challenges due to climate change and fires.

Services

Victorian specialist mental health services are principally provided by two sectors:

1   Clinical mental health.
2   Psychiatric disability rehabilitation support.

Clinical mental health services (older adult, adult, child and adolescent), focus on acute treatment. Psychiatric disability rehabilitation support services provide psychosocial support to people with severe mental health disorders. Most substance use, clinical mental health and psychiatric disability rehabilitation support services are auspiced by either non-government organisations or general hospitals. The Victorian state government, via the Department of Health, allocates funds, sets policy and monitors outcomes for the three sectors. The Australian federal government also has an overarching funding, planning and policy role. While services tend to be primarily state government funded, many have federal government-funded projects braided into their services.

Eastern Hume has 19 substance treatment, clinical mental health and psychiatric disability rehabilitation support agencies with around 220 professionals. Specialist mental health and substance use treatment services are largely provided on an outreach basis from Wangaratta and Wodonga. The substance treatment sector includes two large multi-service counselling organisations and a residential rehabilitation service. Detoxification bed services are usually supplied by local general hospitals or facilities in Melbourne.

The array of community mental health services includes:

➤ Acute psychiatric admission unit.
➤ Adult community mental health agencies in Wangaratta and Wodonga.
➤ Regional older adult and child and adolescent mental health services.
➤ Specialist early psychosis team.
➤ Primary mental health team.

Four Eastern Hume psychiatric disability rehabilitation support services provide community and residential support and rehabilitation to persons with severe mental illness.

Rural challenges

Despite Wangaratta and Wodonga being only a 3–4 hour drive from Melbourne, parts of the region are significantly rural and remote. Many unwanted health outcomes are strongly associated with rural and remote regions. From a mental health–substance use perspective, the most significant of these is that suicide rates increase with increasing rurality, and the significantly elevated rates of hazardous and harmful drinking in rural regions. Rural service delivery challenges include a lack of general and specialist services, travel times and costs and multiple demands on the professional.

CONTEXT
Australian national-level approaches to building mental health–substance use capability

The Australian government's preferred term for mental health–substance use is 'comorbidity'. Since 2003, the Australian government has allocated significant funding to addressing mental health–substance use, primarily in the substance treatment and primary care sectors. Australia, at a national level, has yet to develop a meaningful plan or allocate appropriate resources to developing the mental health sector's recognition of and response to mental health–substance use.

The national comorbidity initiative
The national comorbidity initiative, funded 2003–2011, aims to:
➤ Raise awareness of mental health–substance use amongst health professionals.
➤ Promote examples of good practice.
➤ Support general practitioners and other health professionals to improve treatment outcomes.
➤ Facilitate resources and information for individuals needing care.

The principle programmes and projects to date are summarised in Box 6.1.

BOX 6.1 National comorbidity initiative programmes and projects to date

- **Comorbidity professional development scholarships** to assist substance use and mental health professionals build clinical expertise in the detection and treatment of mental health–substance use.
- **Funding clinical supervision for postgraduate psychologists and social workers** undertaking placements in substance use services.
- **National comorbidity clinical guidelines** focusing on mental health–substance use service delivery in the substance use sector.
- **'Can do' – managing mental health and substance use in general practice** aims to enhance general practitioners' knowledge and skills in identifying and managing mental health–substance use and increase networking between general practitioners and relevant health professionals.
- **Comorbidity service model evaluation** of service delivery models for mental health–substance use treatment in substance use and mental health sectors.
- **PsyCheck** evidence-based treatment programme for substance use services to use with people experiencing depression or anxiety and substance problems.
- **Publications** around various aspects of mental health–substance use.

IMPROVED SERVICES FOR PEOPLE WITH DRUG AND ALCOHOL PROBLEMS AND MENTAL ILLNESS

Funded 2006–2011, the improved services measure aims to build the capacity of substance use services to effectively address and treat mental health–substance use. Individual substance use services were given three-year grants to build their organisation's capacity to respond to the needs of the individual. A second component, the cross-sectoral support and strategic partnership, funds substance use peak bodies to assist services to build partnerships with other health sectors, identify professional development opportunities and undertake service improvement activities.

headspace

Launched in 2006, *headspace* aims to reduce the burden of disease in young people aged 12–25 years caused by mental health and substance use. *headspace* funded the development of 30 'communities of youth services' across Australia – partnerships of health, education and welfare service providers working to reform their response to young people with mental health and substance use issues.

VICTORIAN STATE-LEVEL APPROACHES TO BUILDING MENTAL HEALTH–SUBSTANCE USE CAPABILITY

Of all the Australian states, Victoria has had the longest standing, most substantial investment in achieving better outcomes for persons with mental health–substance use. Victorias' preferred term for mental health–substance use is 'dual diagnosis'. Box 6.2 charts some of the milestones in the evolution of Victoria's responses to mental health–substance use.

BOX 6.2 Evolution of Victoria's responses to mental health–substance use

1998

Substance Use Mental Illness Treatment Team pilot: a partnership of two central policy and planning bodies – the (then) Victorian mental health branch and the drugs policy branch – created the pilot in the western regions of Melbourne and rural Victoria.

2002

Victorian Dual Diagnosis Initiative: the two central planning bodies built on the Substance Use Mental Illness Treatment Team model with the state-wide Victorian Dual Diagnosis Initiative. Around a structure of four metropolitan lead agencies and linked rural professionals the Initiative was given responsibility for capacity building and direct clinical services to agencies and professionals in the three sectors of substance use, community mental health and psychiatric disability rehabilitation support services.

2003

Victorian Dual Diagnosis Initiative augmented by the creation of specialist youth mental health–substance use positions.

2005/06

Victorian Dual Diagnosis Initiative augmented by:
- **Rotations project** – funds mental health or substance use professionals to undertake a 3-month rotation in the 'opposite' sector as core of a 12-month development and education process.

- **State-wide dual diagnosis education and training unit** – developed nationally recognised diploma-level dual diagnosis competencies delivered by a number of education providers via online and in-person delivery.
- **Strengthening psychiatrist support project** – extra specialist mental health–substance use psychiatrist time for the four lead agencies.

2006
- At state government cabinet level a dedicated ministerial position for mental health and drugs created:
- At the central policy and planning level, the former mental health branch and the drugs policy branch merged into the division of mental health and drugs

2007
Policy: state-wide launch of cross-sector 'dual diagnosis: key directions & priorities for service development' policy.[4] The policy contained five service development outcomes, each with key performance indicators and timelines for mental health and substance use services to work towards in developing optimal recognition of and most effective possible responses to the treatment needs of persons experiencing mental health–substance use problems.

EASTERN HUME SYSTEMIC MENTAL HEALTH–SUBSTANCE USE CAPABILITY: A PROGRESS REPORT
Criteria for measuring the development of systemic mental health–substance use capability

The development of systemic mental health–substance use capability is an evolutionary process. Progress in the development of systemic capability may be analysed using criteria such as:
➤ The degree to which the system has developed effective inter-agency relationships.
➤ Agency mental health–substance use capability.
➤ Clinician mental health–substance use capability.
➤ Recognition of mental health–substance use.
➤ Treatment of mental health–substance use.

This section employs these criteria to provide a brief progress report on the current evolution of Eastern Hume systemic mental health–substance use capability.

Degree of system development of effective interagency relationships
The Eastern Hume dual diagnosis group is a long-standing, lively, cross-sector group of managers, clinicians, consumers, carers, portfolio holders and mental health–substance use capacity building professionals, whose aim is to collaboratively build capability to achieve better outcomes for all individuals. The group authored a regional mental health–substance use plan, and member agencies have been successful in funding applications to bring three commonwealth mental health–substance use projects/professionals into the region. Active sub-committees

include a sub-committee that works on developing the range of 'handrails' needed to assist professionals to recognise and respond effectively to persons with mental health–substance use problems. Handrails include policy templates, cross-sector individual treatment plan proformas, position descriptions that include mental health–substance use criteria, treatment guidelines, agreed approaches to collecting data on the prevalence of and outcomes for persons presenting with mental health–substance use.

A central goal is the development of a 'no wrong door' service system. A system in which, when individuals *appear at a facility not qualified to provide some type of needed service, those* [individuals] *are carefully guided to appropriate, cooperating facilities, with follow-up to ensure that* [individuals] *receive proper care*.[3] A dedicated regional project, 'No Wrong Door Phase 2', has made significant ground on this goal through refining and extending an earlier innovative multi-agency protocol, and the use of web technology to assist professionals to make well targeted referrals (*see* www.nowrongdoor.org.au).

Cross-sector systemic orientation days have recently been instigated in which new substance use or mental health professionals, once oriented to their agency, participate in an orientation to the local service system. New professionals visit partner substance use and mental health agencies, and learn about the goals of and their responsibilities in a no wrong door service system.

Agency mental health–substance use capability

All Eastern Hume substance use and mental health agencies have participated in completion of the locally developed '*agency dual diagnosis capability checklists*'.[1] These are comprehensive tools for substance use or mental health agencies to self-assess, reflect on, identify training needs and develop a plan to further develop their agency's levels of mental health–substance use capability (free download/use from www.dualdiagnosis.org.au). All agencies have appointed mental health–substance use portfolio holders – senior clinicians or managers with defined responsibilities around building agency capability.

Service managers are responsible for regular reporting to the Victorian health department on agency's progress in achieving the service development outcomes mandated in the Victorian dual diagnosis policy.[4] All new job descriptions incorporate criteria around required levels of mental health–substance use capability. Professionals preparing for performance reviews can anticipate discussion around their progress in developing their level of mental health–substance use capability. In development are agency screening protocols, amended service descriptions, and mission statements to reflect the agency's recognition of, and responsiveness to the individual experiencing mental health–substance use problems.

Clinician mental health–substance use capability

The Victorian dual diagnosis policy[4] defines '*basic clinician dual diagnosis capability*', as having the capability to screen for and assess, mental health–substance use problems and, '*advanced dual diagnosis capability*', as the ability to screen, assess and treat mental health–substance use disorders. Most Eastern Hume substance use and mental health clinicians are competent/comfortable in screening for mental health–substance use; many are competent in conducting a detailed integrated assessment, and some are competent in providing in-house, one-stop-shop integrated treatment of mental health–substance use problems.

Most professionals are highly attuned to mental health–substance use problems – debates about whether addressing mental health–substance use is core business now rarely occur – and in action around further developing their levels of capability. Most have completed locally designed *'clinician dual diagnosis capability checklists'*[5,6] comprehensive tools to self-assess, reflect on, identify training needs and develop a plan to further develop levels of capability. *Clinician*-level tools, available in substance use or mental health *clinician* specific versions can be downloaded from the 'Tools' section of www.dualdiagnosis.org.au.

Professionals have been exposed to in-house *workshop* trainings since 1998. While workshop training still occurs regularly, we now prioritise professionals undertaking accredited education in the 'opposite' speciality and Hume region department of health has funded large numbers of professionals to undertake accredited training in the 'opposite' speciality – at certificate, graduate diploma and master's levels. In 2009, the Hume Dual Diagnosis Education Collaborative was formed to streamline the delivery of local education and to administer scholarships to Hume professionals.

Recognition of co-occurring mental health–substance use

Local mental health and substance use professionals have received training in detecting and assessing mental health–substance use since 2002. In 2005, Wangaratta mental health services became perhaps the first mental health service in the country to universally screen for mental health–substance use problems using the World Health Organization's comprehensive 'ASSIST' tool.[7] In 2006, gateway substance use service was chosen as one of the Australian implementation sites for the PsyCheck screening and treatment package. All Eastern Hume mental health and substance use services have implemented screening for mental health–substance use disorders. Most Eastern Hume mental health services are now evolving towards conducting routine substance use assessments (rather than screening) as a core component of their routine assessment processes. Similarly, some Eastern Hume substance treatment services are moving towards conducting routine mental state assessments rather than screening for mental health symptoms/disorders.

Treatment of mental health–substance use

The Victorian dual diagnosis policy[4] definition of integrated treatment – *'a clinician treats both the client's substance use and mental health problems. Integrated treatment also occurs when clinicians from separate agencies agree on an individual treatment plan addressing both disorders and then provide treatment. This integration needs to continue after any acute intervention by way of formal interaction and co-operation between agencies in reassessing and treating the client'*[4] – has been promoted strongly in Eastern Hume. The large numbers of professionals who have completed training has built regional capacity to provide one-stop-shop integrated treatment, and examples of both one-stop-shop type and multi-agency integrated treatment are commonplace. Work is progressing on the development of cross-sector individual service plan proformas, and on adopting cross-sector treatment outcome measures.

WHAT WORKS IN ACHIEVING SYSTEMIC CAPABILITY?

Factors that mediate towards sustainable systemic change

This section synthesises learning's from Eastern Hume and Victorian experiences to identify factors that mediate towards sustainable systemic change towards more effective mental health–substance use service delivery.

Taut, readily-deployed rationale

The three foundation stones of mental health–substance use capacity building are:

1 Knowledge of the *prevalence* of mental health–substance use disorders in both general and treated populations.
2 Knowledge of the *harms* strongly associated with mental health–substance use disorders.
3 *Potential* for more effective treatment of 'target' disorders by developing recognition of, and effective responses to, mental health–substance use disorders.

These factors underpin the past two decades of increasing interest in, and resource allocation towards, better addressing mental health–substance use.

These foundations are a potent tool for systems change agents to deploy in influencing professionals, agencies and systems towards change. Many stakeholders remain ambivalent about whether addressing mental health–substance use problems is core business for substance use and mental health professionals. Using appropriate forums to provide information about prevalence and harms can be effective in nudging stakeholders towards action on developing levels of capability. Building stakeholder's appreciation of the potential for more effective treatment of 'target' disorders can serve to engender enthusiasm and to firm up commitment to address mental health–substance use disorders.

Address mental health–substance use at systemic, agency and clinician levels

Addressing mental health–substance use first at a systemic level, (then at agency, then clinician levels), is the most efficient and cost-effective means of coherently, systematically initiating the web of strategies and resource development necessary for significant, sustained system change. Central leadership and direction is a necessary first step to any organisational change process.

A systemic, top-down and bottom-up approach, is critical. Systems that have attempted to address mental health–substance use only at clinician levels – for example with stand alone education and training – have generally had little success due to failure to attend to the range of system-wide strategies, policy and resource development required to align the system with, support and validate, the changed practices.

Charging speciality mental health–substance use professionals with providing direct service for complex needs tends to have little influence on whole agency practice (good practice will not spread osmotically). Relying on a small cohort of professionals to address the needs of individuals with mental health–substance use fails to recognise the prevalence of individuals with mental health–substance use. Focusing on the small cohort of individuals with the most complex needs fails to recognise the potential gains in providing effective responses to the much larger cohorts of individuals with less severe, more easily treated mental health–substance use problems. Similarly, creating specialist mental health–substance use *agencies* fails to recognise prevalence, sends a message that responding to mental health–substance use is only the domain of specialists and has little influence on the whole system's service delivery.

Vision of how the systems will look, feel and function when providing an effective response

Discussions around optimal responses to the challenges posed by mental health–substance use can resemble the fable of six blind men feeling the elephant to satisfy their minds about the nature of the creature. In Saxe's 1881 version[8] the first blind man, feeling the elephant's side proclaimed '*it's very like a wall*'. The second felt the elephant's tusk and said it was like a spear. The third, feeling the trunk, noted the creatures' likeness to a snake. The fourth feeling a knee said it '*is very like a tree*'. The fifth touching an ear decided that the elephant was most like a fan. The sixth, seizing on his tail, averred that the elephant was '*very like a rope*'.

People with mental health–substance use are not a homogeneous group. Given the multiplicity of combinations and severity of problems, the range of treatment needs, and the array of professionals and service settings attempting to meet those needs, there is little surprise that the various stakeholders (individuals, family, carers, professionals, policymakers, researcher), have diverse conceptualisations of:

➤ what the core issues are
➤ how best to address those issues
➤ what the systems will look like when providing effective responses to the needs of the individual.

While there is substantial evidence of the prevalence of and harms strongly associated with mental health–substance use, there is limited evidence available to guide around the nature of the most effective systemic responses.

At first glance, the work involved in agreeing a vision may appear daunting; however, it is an essential task. In the absence of an agreed vision, and plan, the efforts of various stakeholders attempting to improve outcomes for person experiencing mental health–substance use problems will tend to be diffused, and can easily lack coherence, purposefulness, direction, credibility and an evidence base. Across healthcare, there are multiple examples of, often costly, initiatives rolled out funding professionals to address mental health–substance use. Where these initiatives have not evolved into developing a central vision and a plan to achieve it, they have had only limited success.

Having meaningful input into the development of the vision from representatives of all the principle stakeholders, ensures that the vision is realistic and achievable, serves to build ownership and commitment to realising the vision and contributes to the various stakeholders' knowledge, understanding and partnership. The task of engaging the various stakeholders, and facilitating the development of an agreed systemic vision, will usually sit best with central policy and planning bodies. As part of the process of agreeing a vision, and developing a plan to achieve it, it is worthwhile to consider the barriers to developing the system's response to mental health–substance use.

Recognition of the barriers

There are significant barriers[9–15] to developing more effective responses to mental health–substance use. Some of these barriers are listed below.

➤ Professionals, agencies and systems trained and structured to respond only to single disorders/problems.

➤ Service exclusion criteria based on the presence of a mental health–substance use problems.

➤ Stakeholders may lack familiarity with the prevalence, harms, relationships between disorders, and potential for more effective treatment.

➤ Stakeholders may lack knowledge and self-efficacy about effective approaches to addressing mental health–substance use.

➤ In demanding service environments professional's may be '*change-weary and change-wary*'.[9] They may perceive that, implicit in any proposed changes to practice, is an implication that their current practice is 'wrong'.

➤ Lack of understanding of the other treatment system's strengths, constraints and philosophies.

➤ The broader community's lack of knowledge about the interplay of mental health–substance use disorders, and confusion over which disorder is 'primary' and 'secondary'.[15]

➤ Failure to recognise the presence of mental health–substance use problems.

➤ Professionals may perceive addressing mental health–substance use problems as *added work* rather than *more effective work*.

➤ Professionals may lack expertise and confidence in deploying substance use or mental health treatment approaches.

➤ Complexity of individual needs can lead to difficulties in engagement and treatment, professional frustration and the tendency to stigmatisation.

➤ Ineffective mechanisms to achieve clinical care coordination across systems.

➤ Mental health and substance use treatment systems tend to focus scarce resources on treating people with the most severe problems. Treatment for people with the most severe disorders often tends to be high input and less effective in contrast with the – highly prevalent – cohorts of people with less severe mental health–substance use problems where treatment tends to be lower input and more effective. Hence, while the bulk of costs and harms associated with both mental health and substance use problems is attributable to the much larger cohort with less severe mental health–substance use disorders, it is this cohort that most often goes unrecognised or, if recognised, untreated.

➤ Individually mental health and substance use problems are stigmatised. There may be 'compounded stigma' where it is recognised that an individual has both a mental health and a substance use problem. Mental health and substance use service providers are not immune from stigmatising persons with multiple, complex, often difficult to assess and treat disorders.

➤ Tertiary education institutions have been slow to build mental health and substance treatment modalities into most undergraduate healthcare courses despite evidence about the prevalence of persons experiencing mental health and substance use problems across healthcare settings.

An appreciation of the substantial nature of the above barriers mediates towards a longer-term evolutionary perspective around building capability, and informs the selection of strategies in any plan to achieve the vision of how the system will look, feel and function when it is providing more effective responses to people experiencing mental health–substance use problems.

Systemic plans

Typically, in its opening sections, a plan to further develop systemic capability will outline:

➤ the rationale for the system prioritising the development of more effective responses to people experiencing mental health–substance use problems (prevalence, harms, potential)

➤ a discussion around the barriers to the service system providing the most effective possible responses

➤ a vision of how the systems will look, feel and function when providing effective responses to the various cohorts of persons experiencing mental health–substance use problems.

For a plan to be successful, it needs to be crafted with a realistic appraisal of the significant barriers to system change and a strong recognition of the length of time that sustainable system change takes to effect. Hence, a well-honed plan will be written from a longer-term, evolutionary perspective that sends a clear message that central policy and planning bodies prioritise the development of the most effective possible responses and are 'in this for the long haul'.

The plan should provide guidance, around which of the principle treatment sectors – primary care and general practice, specialist mental health and specialist substance use – are assigned primary treatment responsibility for persons experiencing mental health–substance use problems. The most well known device to effect this is the USA's four-quadrant model.[16] However, the three-level schema in the Victorian dual diagnosis policy,[4] is also worth reviewing. Assigning broad treatment responsibility for the various cohorts is a step towards developing a 'no wrong door' system – the guidance in such a model is valued by front-line professionals.

To be effective in achieving sustainable system change a plan must contain clear, achievable, explicit goals. Given:

➤ the range of interpretations about what is best practice

➤ the barriers to the provision of the most effective possible responses

➤ that some healthcare providers – perhaps besieged with competing priorities and lacking familiarity with mental health–substance use prevalence, harms and potential – remain precontemplative about addressing mental health–substance use; it is necessary that the goals are clearly and explicitly stated and, ideally, are accompanied by:

— key performance indicators
— clear statements of responsibility for achieving goals
— timelines for their achievement
— reporting mechanisms.

It could be argued that this degree of specificity and accountability may engender resistance from those charged with achieving and reporting on the goals. Following the roll-out of the Victorian policy, the perception has been that front-line professionals and service professionals feel supported by, and have welcomed clear direction from, central policy and planning bodies. The risk of provoking resistance in professionals and service professionals may be ameliorated by promoting the systemic plan in a motivational fashion, for example by facilitators at forums introducing the plan providing opportunities for participants to reflect on the prevalence, harms and potentials around mental health–substance use in the particular service setting, in which, the participant works.

Plans should define and prioritise the further development of capability – at both clinician and agency levels. Victorian dual diagnosis policy definitions of 'dual diagnosis capability' were included in the preceding section of this chapter.

Alongside a clear statement that addressing mental health–substance use, is core business the plan should prioritise the development of the system's ability to detect and assess mental health–substance use disorders. The plan should provide an operational, achievable definition of 'integrated treatment' alongside central policy guidance about the systems degree of support for the goal of routine integrated treatment. In the USA, the federal Substance Abuse Mental Health Services Administration body, has robustly promoted integrated treatment of low-prevalence mental health problems type mental health–substance use as one of six evidence-based practices identified for mental health services.[17] The Victorian policy[4] prioritises integrated treatment defining it as *either a single professional or agency treating both disorders, or multiple agency involvement with the agencies collaborating on the development of a single individual service plan, and having ongoing interagency communication as the individual's treatment progresses.*

The final, essential component of an effective plan is the statement of a 'no wrong door' goal. Challenges for service systems in the achievement of 'no wrong door' goals, include aligning intake criteria and processes with a 'no wrong door' policy, building flexible interagency relationships and referral pathways, and professional orientation towards achieving a 'no wrong door' service system.

Handrails

Systems and agencies addressing their responses to mental health–substance use often tend as a first, sometimes only, strategy to focus on providing education and training. Education provided in the absence of a system wide change process – a process that includes the motivational deployment of a web of strategies and supports to changed practice – will almost certainly be a waste of resources.

Professionals may return from the training enthused about instituting screening and more integrated treatment only to find that key professionals within their agency do not understand – perhaps oppose – the changes to practice, and that the tools and handrails necessary to support changed practice are not available.

Some of the tools and handrails that need to be created or modified to align the services with the changed practices, and support professionals in better recognition of, and more effective responses, include:
➤ Clinical treatment guidelines.
➤ Agency descriptions and mission statements.
➤ Job descriptions – to incorporate criteria around required levels of mental health–substance use capability.
➤ Revised professional orientation manuals and procedures.
➤ Policy and protocols – including:
  — *no wrong door policy*
  — *secondary consultation* policies and proformas – a diversity of healthcare services are mandated to provide secondary consultation as core business but few professionals or services are supported in this by clear policy guidance and education around the responsibilities and skills involved in seeking, receiving or providing effective secondary consultation. There is potential for contributing to a 'no wrong door' service system, and more effective use of scarce healthcare resources, in providing clear policy guidance around secondary consultation and training to professionals in the skills required to seek and provide effective secondary consultations
  — *protocols between substance use and mental health agencies* that provide guidance to professionals about how the agencies can work together most effectively in the interests of the individual. Such protocols typically assign broad treatment responsibility for the various cohorts of persons experiencing mental health–substance use problems, and outline treatment pathways between services, the priority of interagency cooperation, and detail dispute resolution mechanisms
  — *screening and assessment protocol.*
➤ Tools for self assessing agency levels of mental health–substance use capability–some of the tools that agencies may consider for this purpose are:
  — checklists – agency Dual Diagnosis capability[1,2]
  — compass – comorbidity use programme audit and self-survey for behavioural health services[18]
  — dual diagnosis capability in substance use treatment index[19]
  — dual diagnosis capability in mental health treatment.[20]
➤ Tools for self assessing professional levels of mental health–substance use capability:
  — checklists – mental health–substance use capability – clinician versions[5,6]
  — codecat – Co-occurring Disorders Educational Competency Assessment Tool.[21]
➤ Screening and assessment proformas – for detecting, assessing and treatment planning around mental health–substance use problems:

➤ Cross-sector individual treatment plan proformas[22] – needed for situations where the individual's best interests are served by having multiple agencies involved. Proformas should assist professionals and individuals to document what goals will be addressed by which agency; permission for, methods, timing and frequency of communication between the professional in the involved agencies, outcome measures and mechanisms for data collection.

If the process of creating and/or refining these handrails can be commenced in advance of the deployment of education and training this serves to build local investment in the change process, reinforce the direction the system is moving in, and place necessary tools in the hands of the professionals delivering treatment.

Education and training

The timing of education and training delivery is critical. If imposed when professionals are largely precontemplative about addressing their responses, it is likely to have little influence on service delivery and may even engender resistance (by introducing change talk before the 'individual' discerns any need for change). Conversely, by virtue of providing realistic information and feedback, it may also serve to nudge stakeholders from precontemplative to contemplative. Once professionals, agencies and systems are enthusiastic about developing their levels of capability, it is critical that there is a range of coherent, quality education and training options to meet stakeholders varying learning styles and needs.

It is necessary to use a range of strategies to make it as easier for professionals to participate in education and training. Scholarships, e-learning, study leave, offering both in-house workshops and accredited courses are all-necessary to educate professionals towards new practices. Education needs to be tailored specifically to the differing needs of substance use and mental health professionals, and joint education around some topics, as another strategy to build links and working relationships between the sectors. Education and training packages need to be developed around the specific needs of the individual, family and carers. Clinical supervision should be available to reinforce, and work with the professional during and following education and training.

In Victoria, a 'best buy' by central policy and planning bodies was investing in a statewide mental health–substance use education and training unit. With a small staff and within a short time, this unit developed and delivered accredited courses and curricula for a range of health related undergraduate and postgraduate courses. The unit has deployed a host of innovative activities that have substantially contributed to the quality and consistency of education and training delivery. Victoria has also invested heavily in the 'rotations project' in which, interested mental health or substance use professionals are funded to spend a 3-month rotation in the 'other' sector as the hub of a 12-month development process that includes accredited mental health–substance use education.

Change agents

For a plan to succeed the system must have persons whose assigned roles include achieving the plan goals. Reporting responsibilities for key performance indicators in a systemic plan is most efficiently assigned to the managers of individual agencies. This strategy does not impose a new cost on the system, and ensures that managers are familiar with and invested in achieving the plan's goals. Managers are the predominant culture setters in any organisation and their enthusiasm for any change process is essential.

Another low-cost strategy is to centrally mandate that each agency in the system assign a professional the role of mental health–substance use portfolio holder. Ideally, the portfolio holder will be a senior person who is also an 'opinion leader' within the organisation. Remuneration for taking on this role could take the form of a reduction in caseload, seniority or financial remuneration.

If the system has sufficient resources, it may consider the deployment of a specialist mental health–substance use workforce. The trajectory of such workforces tends to be from an initial emphasis on direct service delivery or 'co-case management' for persons with complex needs to an emphasis on a diverse range of capacity building strategies necessary to sustainably change practice.

Partnerships

Effective partnerships are both a goal of, and a method of, achieving a mental health–substance use capable service system. Perhaps the most effective systemic change agents are partnerships of agencies within a system or sub-system. Ideally, such groups will include the individual experiencing mental health–substance use problems, the family and or carer representatives, managers of individual agencies, portfolio holders and specialist mental health–substance use professionals. Significant diverse gains and synergies occur once a system has successfully formed a cross-sector alliance of local agencies interested in cooperatively achieving a plan to enhance systemic capability.

Prior to the formation of the Eastern Hume Dual Diagnosis Service, most mental health–substance use capability developments were attributable to local specialist mental health–substance use professionals. Since the formation of this service a number of cross-sector, cross-agency initiatives have occurred without any involvement by local specialist mental health–substance use professionals.

Resource allocation

How much, or how little, a change process costs in financial terms is up to the system that designs it. If the system is successful in building professionals and agencies appreciation of the prevalence, harms and enthusiasm for the potential associated with mental health–substance use then it will have tapped into the most powerful, no extra cost resource towards a capable service system. A collaboratively developed, agreed, systemic vision costs very little to develop; a well-crafted plan only slightly more.

Many of the handrails to assist professionals in changed practices can be developed at little cost. There are numerous templates available. Creating a central mental health–substance use education and training unit is clearly a 'best-buy'. Attributing reporting responsibilities to service managers is a negligible-cost, powerful strategy towards increasing mental health–substance use capability. There are some costs involved in changing professional's position descriptions to incorporate a mental health–substance use portfolio holder role and more substantial costs, albeit substantial rewards, in creating dedicated capacity-building roles.

Multiple strategies – sustained efforts

In 2005, one study,[23] drew on decades of experience in addressing mental health–substance use at individual, family, carer, professional, agency, state and national levels to note that:

> *There are no magic bullets for changing provider behaviour in health care. What does appear clear is that combining multiple strategies to overcome challenges is more likely to be effective than using just one intervention . . .* [and] *In studies of practice change intensity of effort appears directly related to success.*[23]

Building a healthcare system's capacity to recognise and respond effectively to the various cohorts of persons experiencing mental health–substance use problems is long-term work. However, careful planning and attention to the elements described above can considerably expedite this process.

CONCLUSION

The experience in Eastern Hume has been that it is possible to influence professionals, agencies and systems to evolve towards sustainable mental health–substance use capability. Processes aimed at building systemic capability are more likely to be successful if they are built on an agreed vision of how a system will look, feel and function, when providing more effective treatment to the individual experiencing mental health–substance use problems.

Plans to achieve that vision need to be developed with recognition of the multiple barriers to successful system change, and incorporate a web of complementary, carefully chosen strategies with clear attribution of responsibility and timelines for their achievement. Effective cross-sector partnerships are a fundamental goal for any systemic mental health–substance use capability development process, and a vital method to achieve systemic capability. It is possible to attend to the essentials required to develop systemic mental health–substance use capability without significant resource allocation.

POST-READING EXERCISE 6.1

Time: 50 minutes
- Review the plan that you developed in the Pre-Reading Exercise 6.1, using the 'agency dual diagnosis capability checklist'.
- Would you amend any of your plan based on the material discussed in this chapter?
- What are the three most influential strategies you could deploy to influence your agency's levels of mental health–substance use capability?

REFERENCES

1 Croton G. *Checklist: dual diagnosis capability – agency/service level (Victorian version)*. Northeast Health Wangaratta; 2008. Available at: www.dualdiagnosis.org.au/home/index.php?option=com_docman&task=doc_details&gid=34&Itemid=27 (accessed 7 June 2010).

2 Croton G. *Checklist: dual diagnosis capability – agency/service level (non-Victorian version)*. Northeast Health Wangaratta; 2008. Available at: www.dualdiagnosis.org.au/home/index.php?option=com_docman&task=doc_details&gid=33&Itemid=27 (accessed 7 June 2010).

3 Center for Substance Abuse Treatment. *Substance Abuse Treatment for Persons with Co-occurring Disorders: treatment improvement protocol (tip) series 42*. Department of Health and Human Services Publication no. (SMA) 05–3992. Rockville, MD: Substance Abuse and Mental Health Service Administration; 2005.

4 Victorian Government. *Dual Diagnosis: key directions and priorities for service development*. Victorian Government Department of Human Services, Melbourne, VIC: Available from www.health.vic.gov.au/mentalhealth/dualdiagnosis/ or www.health.vic.gov.au/drugservices/pubs/dual_diagnosis.htm (accessed 7 June 2010).

5 Croton G. *Checklist: dual diagnosis capability – alcohol, tobacco and other drug workers*. Northeast Health Wangaratta: 2008. Available at: www.dualdiagnosis.org.au/home/index.php?option=com_docman&task=doc_details&gid=35&Itemid=27 (accessed 7 June 2010).

6 Croton G. *Checklist: dual diagnosis capability – clinical mental health workers*. Northeast Health Wangaratta; 2008. Available at: www.dualdiagnosis.org.au/home/indexphp?option=com_docman&task=doc_details&gid=36&Itemid=27 (accessed 7 June 2010).

7 Henry-Edwards S, Humeniuk R, Ali R, *et al*. *The Alcohol, Smoking and Substance Involvement Screening Test (ASSIST): guidelines for use in primary care* (draft version 1.1 for field-testing). Geneva: World Health Organization; 2003. Available at: www.who.int/substance_abuse activities/assist_v3_english.pdf (accessed 7 June 2010).

8 Saxe J. *The Poems of John Godfrey Saxe*. Highgate Edition, Boston, MA: Houghton, Mifflin & Co.; 1881.

9 Croton G. *Australian Treatment System's Recognition of and Response to Co-occurring Mental Health and Substance Use Disorders*. Senate Mental Health Inquiry Submission. Northeast Health Wangaratta; 2005. Available at: www.dualdiagnosis.org.au/home/index.php?option=com_docman&task=doc_details&gid=4&Itemid=27 (accessed 7 June 2010).

10 Addiction Technology Transfer Centers. *The Change Book: a blueprint for technology transfer*. Center for Substance Abuse Treatment. Rockville, MD: Substance Abuse and Mental Health Service Administration; 2004. Available at: www.nattc.org/respubs/changebook.html (accessed 7 June 2010).

11 Zweben J. Severely and persistently mentally ill substance abusers: clinical and policy issues. *J Psychoactive Drugs*. 2000; **32**: 383–9.

12 Watkins K, Burnham A, Kung F-U, *et al*. A national survey of care for persons with co-occurring mental and substance use disorders. *Psychiatr Serv*. 2001; **52**: 1062–8.

13 Todd F, Sellman D, Robertson P. Barriers to optimal care for patients with coexisting substance use and mental health disorders. *Aust N Z J Psychiatry*. 2002; **36**: 792–9.

14 Kavanagh D, Greenaway I, Jenner I, *et al*. Contrasting views and experiences of health professionals on the management of comorbid substance use and mental health disorders. *Aust N Z J Psychiatry*. 2000; **34**: 279–89.

15 Drake R, Essock S, Shaner A, *et al.* Implementing dual diagnosis services for clients with severe mental illness. *Psychiatr Serv.* 2001; **52**: 179–82.

16 National Association of State Mental Health Program Directors, National Association of State Alcohol and Drug Abuse Directors. *National Dialogue on Co-occurring Mental Health and Substance Abuse Disorders.* 1998. Cited in: Center for Substance Abuse Treatment. *Definitions and Terms Relating to Co-occurring Disorders.* COCE Overview Paper 1. DHHS Publication no. (SMA) 07–4163. Rockville, MD: Substance Abuse and Mental Health Services Administation and Centre for Mental Health Services; 2007. Available at: http:// coce.samhsa.gov/cod_resources/PDF/OP1-DefinitionsandTerms-8-13-07.pdf (accessed 10 August 2010).

17 Substance Abuse and Mental Health Service Administration. *Evidence-based Practices: shaping mental health services toward recovery implementation – resource kit user's guide*; 2005. Available at: mentalhealth.samhsa.gov/cmhs/communitysupport/toolkits/cooccurring/ (accessed 7 June 2010).

18 Minkoff K, Cline C. *Comorbidity Program Audit and Self-survey for Behavioral Health Services.* Co-occurring Disorders Services Enhancement Toolkit: tool number 5; 2001. Available at: www.zialogic.org/tool_no__5.htm (accessed 7 June 2010).

19 McGovern MP, Girard J, Kincaid R, *et al. A Toolkit for Enhancing Addiction Only Service (AOS) Programs and Dual Diagnosis Capable (DDC) Programs.* The Dual Diagnosis Capability in Addiction Treatment (DDCAT) Index; 2010. Available at: www.dartmouth. edu/~prc/page18/page18.html (accessed 7 June 2010).

20 Gotham, Brown J, Comaty J, *et al. Dual Diagnosis Capability in Mental Health Treatment (DDCMHT).* Version 3.2; 2007. Available at: www.dartmouth.edu/~prc/page18/page18. html (accessed 7 June 2010).

21 Minkoff K, Cline C. *CODECAT: Co-occurring disorders educational competency assessment tool.* Co-occurring disorders services enhancement toolkit – tool number 3. Available at: www.zialogic.org/tool_no__3.htm (accessed 7 June 2010)

22 Croton G. *Screening for and Assessment of Co-occurring Substance Use and Mental Health Disorders by Alcohol and Other Drug and Mental Health Services.* Victorian Dual Diagnosis Initiative Advisory Group, Victoria; 2007. Available at: www.dualdiagnosis.org.au/home/ index.php?option=com_docman&task=doc_details&gid=23&Itemid=27 (accessed 7 June 2010).

23 Torrey WC, Gorman PG. Closing the gap between what services are and what they could be. In: Drake R, Merrens M, Lynde D, editors. *Evidence-based Mental Health Practice: a textbook.* New York: WW Norton; 2005.

TO LEARN MORE
Australian national-level responses to mental health–substance use
National Comorbidity Initiative
- www.health.gov.au/internet/mentalhealth/publishing.nsf/content/national-comorbidity-initiative-2

The Improved Services measure
- www.health.gov.au/internet/mentalhealth/publishing.nsf/content/drug-alcohol-mental-illness-1
- www.comorbidity.org.au/

headspace
- www.headspace.org.au/

Comorbidity professional development scholarships
- www.nceta.flinders.edu.au/projects/comorbidity.html

'Can Do': managing mental health and substance use in general practice
- www.agpncando.com/

Comprehensive Continuous Integrated System of Care Model
- www.zialogic.org/
- www.kenminkoff.com/

Screening for mental health–substance use
PsyCheck
- www.psycheck.org.au/

WHO 'ASSIST' tool
- www.who.int/substance_abuse/activities/assist/en/index.html

Tools for assessing agency levels of mental health–substance use capability
Checklists: service level dual diagnosis capability – agency (Victorian or non-Victorian versions)
- www.dualdiagnosis.org.au

Comorbidity program audit and self-survey for behavioral health services
- www.zialogic.org/

Dual diagnosis capability in addiction treatment index
- www.dartmouth.edu/~prc/page18/page18.html

Dual diagnosis capability in mental health treatment
- www.dartmouth.edu/~prc/page18/page18.html

Integrated dual disorders treatment fidelity scale
- http://mentalhealth.samhsa.gov/cmhs/communitysupport/toolkits/cooccurring/

Tools for assessing clinician levels of mental health–substance use capability
Checklists: dual diagnosis capability – clinician (substance use or mental health clinician versions)
- www.dualdiagnosis.org.au

Co-occurring Disorders Educational Competency Assessment Tool
- www.zialogic.org/

Victorian and Eastern Hume responses to mental health–substance use

Victorian dual diagnosis policy

- www.health.vic.gov.au/mentalhealth/dualdiagnosis/
- www.health.vic.gov.au/drugservices/pubs/dual_diagnosis.htm

Dual Diagnosis Australia and New Zealand

- www.dualdiagnosis.org.au

Dual Diagnosis Support Victoria

- http://dualdiagnosis.ning.com/

No Wrong Door phase 2

- www.nowrongdoor.org.au

CHAPTER 7

Developing and evaluating innovative community programmes

Diana PK Roeg and Theo JM Kuunders

PRE-READING EXERCISE 7.1 (ANSWERS ON P. 109)

Time: 30 minutes

1   What is intensive community-based care? Do you know of some examples in your own surroundings? Try to think of a number of its possible characteristics and write down a short description.
2   Intensive community-based care was developed about 50 years ago.
  * Why?
  * For whom?

HOW IT STARTED
Anti-psychiatry

Psychiatric hospitals provided medical treatment in combination with asylum for decennia. Individuals (i.e. mentally disordered, substance use problems and anti-social persons) lived, worked, ate, slept and spent their free time on the terrain of the hospital.[1,2] Most people in a psychiatric hospital, stayed there for the rest of their lives. Reintegration appeared to be very hard. Some said that living in hospital had 'debilitated' these individuals and made them passive.[1,3]

About 50 years ago, increasing numbers of individuals and psychiatrists began to agitate against the 'medical model' of mental healthcare, in which mental illness was primarily viewed as a biological phenomenon. They wanted mental health-care to pay more attention to the social life of the individual.[4] These ideas gained increasing support and in the 1960s, had grown into a movement now known as 'anti-psychiatry'.[2] The mental healthcare system changed internationally, and community-based alternatives for the psychiatric hospital were developed.[3,5] Wards were modernised and new ambulant services established. Individuals were 'trained' to live in the community, family support systems were created, as well as houses for supported living. It was no longer necessary to live in a hospital to receive treat-ment.[1] In the 1980s–1990s, emphasis on extending methods for social psychiatric care (sheltered residences and home-treatment), went together with economic goals of cost control in care institutions.[6,7]

Outgoing

The living circumstances for most individuals improved enormously. However, for some, 'living in the community' appeared too much and too soon. A group of people became deprived and marginalised. These individuals had limited sickness awareness, could not manage daily living (eating healthy, arranging health assurance, making money or finding accommodation), and could not, or would not, find their way to the appropriate services. Critics even suggested that the individual had simply been moved from the 'back wards' of the hospital to the 'back alleys' of the community.[8] Fragmentised healthcare system contributed to this problem. It was not suited for people with complex or combined problems, leading to unreached and 'revolving door' and high drop-out figures.[9,10]

Outreaching and intensive variants of mental healthcare services came into existence to support this complex target population. These services were characterised by the outgoing approach of professionals, high frequent contact, and care coordination.[11,12] They were *'packages of elements that guide the professional in his/her work with individuals',*[13] also referred to as healthcare programmes. A general term, covering all types of programmes, is intensive community-based care.[1,3,14,15]

TYPES OF PROGRAMMES

Introduced in the 1970s, case management coordinated a person's healthcare to provide stability and continuity, while Training in Community Living extended this concept to include treating people in their own environment.[12] Many variants on these programmes appeared. One study,[15] distinguished six types of programme models:

1 broker service
2 clinical case management
3 assertive community treatment
4 intensive case management
5 strengths
6 rehabilitation.

All intensive community-based care programmes are made up of the following components:[11]

➤ **Ideologies**: reflect moral perceptions of how psychiatric and substance use problems should be approached and treated (e.g. the individual needs to live as much as possible within the community; should be supported to find appropriate services; commitment of professionals should be continuous).

➤ **Objectives**: main objectives are engagement, continuity of care, reduction of days in the hospital, cost reduction and improvement of quality of life.[15,16]

➤ **Functions**: included in a particular programme they vary according to the level of model comprehensiveness. Basic functions are outreach, assessment, case planning, and referral or direct services provision. The more comprehensive models include, case finding (i.e. tracing potential individuals), establishing a relationship, rehabilitation services, and advocacy.

➤ **Structure**: refers to the way things are organised and how care is linked within existing healthcare services. Relevant components include, team structure, inter-organisational cooperation, task division, and coordination. In practice, we often see mixed-model implementations. In the UK, these are known as Assertive Outreach Teams and Community Mental Health Teams. In the Netherlands, there are interferential care teams (inter-organisational), and teams that work with adaptations of the assertive community treatment model.

IMPLEMENTING A PROGRAMME: TOOLS FOR MANAGERS

There are many programmes, but which is most effective? It is proven that intensive community-based care has a number of advantages over 'care as usual' – reduction of hospital use; increase of retention in treatment; increased satisfaction.[17] However, we do not know whether positive effects may be due to a whole programme or simply due to one or two individual *programme components* (such as, increased attention and time spent by professionals).[18] Moreover, the context in which a programme is implemented seems to play a role. Some authors suggest that by comparing programmes in different regions and countries, the type and quality of services available in the direct surroundings of an intensive community-based care programme influence the necessity of certain programme components and determine the organisational form of the programme.[1,19] For instance, the assertive community treatment model showed good results in the US, mainly on reduction of hospitalisation and individual satisfaction but in the UK, it did not contribute much to the care as usual.[19] Some say it is because 'standard' care in Europe already contains many elements of intensive community-based care.[20]

CASE DESCRIPTION OF AN INTENSIVE COMMUNITY-BASED CARE APPROACH

> Liz, 45, lives alone in a rented house. Her social housing organisation reports behavioural nuisance and calls for help at the counter for inter-ferential care. Social housing considers removing her (lawfully) from the house, because she did not answer after several written warnings. Liz is awake at night, goes outside and howls like a wolf. Her neighbours cannot stand this. There is a long history of complaints about her behaviour. The professional, Susan, collects information about Liz and finds that she is diagnosed with schizophrenic disorder and had previous enforced psychiatric treatment. After unfruitful attempts to contact her (Liz keeps her door closed), Susan decides to stand watch in the street at night. She manages to address Liz and tells her that people are concerned. Searching for an entrance, Susan mentions that Liz's general practitioner is concerned that her medication should be prolonged. Liz accepts Susan's approach. Inside her house they have a conversation. Susan finds that former admissions in a local psychiatric ward were traumatic. Besides isolated treatment, Liz received probe feeding against her will. She has no

intention at all to ever accept treatment again at the institution. With this information, Susan understands why Liz holds back. At the same time, the threat of being removed from her home has to be discussed. In subsequent appointments, Susan slowly gains Liz's trust. After three months, Susan explains the binding conditions set by the housing organisation. If Liz wants to stay in her home, she will have to accept regular guidance of a professional. This is considered a coercive (by contract) procedure called 'last chance policy'. The individual needs to comprehend that there is something to gain; in exchange, Liz has to commit to certain treatment. From this point, Susan can focus on negotiations to identify the best circumstances for Liz, and facilitate her compliance so Liz will work with the contract. One important condition for Liz is that she will not have to go to the former psychiatric hospital for regular appointments. To Susan this sounds very reasonable. However, in spite of clear agreement between Susan and the care continuator, the regular team decides that Liz should overcome her fear for the past and accept appointments at the psychiatric hospital.

This demonstrates a successful approach in supporting the individual (Liz) and reducing thresholds for the acceptance of care as a primary goal. However, it demonstrates how the professional (Susan) can be frustrated when this goal is no longer recognised by care continuators and the therapeutic relationship is lost.

PROVIDING INTENSIVE CARE: TOOLS FOR THE PROFESSIONAL
Job description

Intensive community-based care is, in principle, based on voluntary commitment. However, due to the persuasive character, it can vary from voluntary to compulsive care. On a continuum from voluntary to compulsory, intensive community-based care can be placed somewhere in the middle (*see* Figure 7.1). It includes help that is uninvited but is later accepted when offered or an approach where actual persuasion is needed.[21] Motivation is key and requires that regardless of the type of intensive community-based care, it must try to accommodate individual needs with the services being offered.

KEY POINT 7.1

Quote from a professional: *You cannot change 'care avoiders', you can only change the way to treat them.*

Functions included in the healthcare process of an intensive community-based care programme depend on the choices made by management during implementation of the programme. Relevant functions include:[11,22,23]

➤ **Case finding**: searching for potential individuals experiencing problems. This can be done by fieldwork, or by making use of a report system: persons or

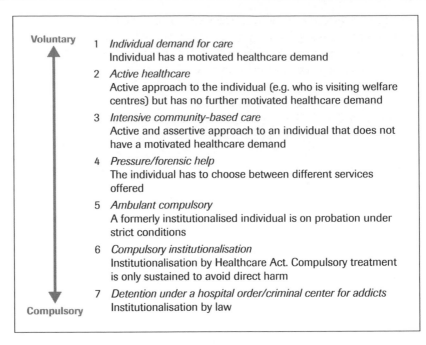

FIGURE 7.1 Interferential care on a continuum of voluntariness[21]

institutes that can contact the team when they are worried or experiencing nuisance.

➤ **Assessment**: identifying the main problem areas. This can be done in conversation with the individual themselves, and via their network (parents, partner, neighbours, other professionals, property owner, etc.).

➤ **Personal working relationship and sustaining contact**: individual personal (working) relation is the base for further services. Trust needs to be built and maintained. This is especially important, as the services are not coercive but voluntary. The best practice strategy is to start simple and move slowly: start for instance with chatting over coffee. Let the person feel he/she is in charge. Next step is sustaining contact.

➤ **Advocacy**: includes the contact with others as spokesperson for the individual. 'Others' can be relevant institutes (e.g. social services, housing corporations) or the individuals' network.

➤ **Quarter mastering**: creating acceptance in the neighbourhood.

➤ **Healthcare planning**: focusing services provided. It includes a number of tasks, discussed with the individual, that need to be undertaken.

➤ **Linking and coordination**: securing proper facilities and services for the individual and making sure use is made of these.

➤ **Rehabilitation**: is helping the individual 'live in the community' as autonomously as possible.

➤ **Outreach**: an important part of intensive community-based care. Contact with the individual is often within her/his home environment.

➤ **Methodologies**: include direct services. They can include all relevant methodologies available. Often it depends on the professionals' background/ education and additional training.

➤ **Pressure/coercion/temptation:** a main characteristic of this type of care and refers to strategies to encourage the individual to accept help that is offered.

➤ **Closing:** ending individual/professional relationship. Involvement with the individual can create dependency, on both sides. Therefore, it is important to make clear at the outset that the involvement may only be temporary and that other professionals may be involved. This reduces expectation, aids the individual in preparation for closure with that professional, and prepare for the possible intervention by other professionals. This can also include a referral. However, some individual need a long-lasting contact with a team to prevent relapse.

➤ **Follow-up:** checking post closure to make sure the situation remains stable.

KEY POINT 7.2

Quote from a professional: *The job is not done when a patient is transferred to regular care; for many, community-based care is a lifetime necessity.*

Provider characteristics

Research demonstrates that professionals need to have specific characteristics. Years of experience and belief in efficacy of the intervention, are proven to contribute to service linkage and outreach activities.[24] Although, after more than 15 years experience, professionals actually performed *less* of these central activities with each additional year of experience.

One stretches the importance of the personal make up, such as readiness to break frontiers, an open mind and strategic bargain capacities.[25,26] Other capacities include:

➤ tailoring care to individual needs
➤ being capable of managing a crisis situation
➤ being gently persistent.

Not having the necessary characteristics might be a risk factor for burnout when working in an intensive community-based care team. Professionals have to manage individuals with mental health–substance use problems who can be difficult-to-engage and have high severity of clinical and social problems. A London study showed that although professionals are fairly satisfied with their jobs, and most are not experiencing high levels of burnout, just over one-third of the teams have potential for the 'emotional exhaustion' component of burnout.[14] However, the organisation also plays an important role:

➤ being well resourced (e.g. availability of a psychiatrist; of dedicated beds; extent to which professionals' work outside usual office hours) seem to work preventively
➤ being well trained (e.g. in techniques for outreach; mental health–substance

use problems; working with the individuals family; advising on housing and benefits) seem to work preventively as well
➤ length of service in current post is associated with more burnout, a factor also mentioned in other research (*see* Chapters 10,11 and 12).[14,25,26]

Box 7.1 summarises the personal characteristics needed for professionals in the intensive community-based care.

BOX 7.1 Relevant provider characteristics

- Being 'a type' for the job (e.g. having an open mind and bargain strategies, being persistent).
- Believing in the efficacy of the intervention.
- Being well trained (e.g. techniques for outreach, mental health–substance use, working with the individual's families, giving advice on housing and benefits).
- Having some years of experience, though not staying too long on the same post.

Supporting the professional teams

To perform tasks in intensive community-based care successfully, professionals need sound conditions on two levels:

1 professional characteristics need to be coached by creating the necessary working environment on a practical and functional level of professional team- and self-reflection
2 at an institutional level, create recognition within the organisation for the importance of continuity of the community-based outlines.

Methods of reflection, such as Socratic conversation method, offer a scholarly approach to peer case review that identifies and analyses quality-of-care issues in response to a question about nursing care. The comprehensive method provides a structured format that critically examines:
➤ untoward events
➤ generates awareness of gaps in care from a systems perspective
➤ ensures action planning focused on legitimate root causes
➤ stimulates performance improvement initiatives
➤ provides an opportunity to share learning within the professional team.[27]

The reflexive question-and-answer process is moved from a one-on-one dialogue to a dialogue between multiple participants. The method is:
➤ inductive
➤ rooted in the experiences of the participants
➤ invites the individual to look beyond practical care issues
➤ explore basic (moral) convictions.

The method can enforce the team's sense of shared responsibility.

Coaching professional teams at institutional level requires harmonisation of the organisation with the general goals of community-based care: persistence, belief in the same care methods and active outreaching approaches. Often professionals are frustrated after a successful intensive and persuasive approach. Shortly after having transferred the (formerly unwilling) person to a regular care unit, the care relation has ended due to 'insufficient motivation' on the individuals behalf. The risk of exhaustion and disappointment for professionals grows proportional with the inadequacy of institutional accommodation to specific individual complex needs.

EVALUATION OF CARE

How to

Evaluation determines effective services. This can be done on individual one-to-one/person-to-person level, for instance in a conversation with the individual or in a team meeting with colleagues. However, when evaluating the programme, information from larger groups of individuals experiencing problems, and systematic measurement is needed. For a sound robust study, the following is needed:

1 **Detailed description of the programme itself, including all components.** Various instruments are developed for programme description.[28–30] A good description is needed to explain the effects and to support replication. It is helpful to compare programmes.

2 **A pre- and post-measurement of each individual – and additionally a follow-up measurement to assess long-term effects.** Validated instruments for such measurements are required. It is relevant to use outcome measures that match the objectives of the programme. This can vary from reduction of mental health and or substance use symptoms, to enlarged engagement in healthcare. Measurement takes time – time well spent. When organised effectively, results can be used directly in individual contacts (e.g. to monitor progress). The results help the team to professionalise services provided. Useful measurement instruments are those developed for routine outcome measurement: they are short, practical and validated. Examples include:
   — engagement measure – engagement[31]
   — Health of the Nation Outcome Scales – problem severity[32]
   — Kennedy Axis V – problem severity[33]
   — Manchester Short Assessment of Quality of Life – perceived quality of life.[34]

3 **A control group that receives no care or 'care as usual' and randomised assignment.** A control group is needed to check whether the services of your team have other consequences (better results), than doing nothing or providing regular healthcare services. Randomised assignment is needed to ensure the individuals' characteristics (like problem severity) are comparable in both groups. In community-based care, it is difficult to maintain a control group, as people can be avoiding. The only way to get in contact, or to commit to services, is intensive community-based care. Fortunately, without control group and randomisation, evaluation can be undertaken – this is termed 'quasi-experimental'.

The role of professionals and the individual's records for evaluation of care

Professionals value records of data because they offer a clear insight in the individual care process. The record structures service activities (e.g. perform job responsibilities), and provides actual information in case of transfer. A main concern for the professional is a quick supply of information on the individuals' network:

➤ Who is involved?
➤ Has care been received recently?
➤ Are there any pitfalls to take into account?

The professional's qualitative records serve other purposes than quantitative evaluation. Professionals will acknowledge the importance of effective evaluation. However, practical experience demonstrates that demands for registration, and recording systems for evaluation, should not become too complex. Special attention should be given to the crucial role of the professional in collecting the necessary evaluation data. Their motivation to contribute to evaluation of care is maximised by having a perspective on how outcome data could be used to improve and professionalise the primary care process. Since learning from experience is viewed as an important strategy for health professionals, who often embrace lifelong learning, their engagement in evaluation of care is associated with the improvement of the quality of direct patient care and stimulating personal and professional growth. Closing the gap between theory and practice requires consideration with this learning strategy.[35]

CONCLUSION

Intensive community-based care is an alternative for the psychiatric hospital and is aimed at persons with severe mental health–substance use problems that, by themselves, do not reach healthcare. It is characterised by an outgoing approach of professionals, high frequent contact, and care coordination. Services are provided in the person's own environment and training is available to aid community living. There are several model programmes described to use as an example for them who want to implement an intensive community-based care programme. Most important is to tune the content of the new programme to the 'standard care' already available locally. For professionals, the functions of intensive community-based care were presented, as well as personal characteristics, education and resources that are needed to do the job. Intensive community-based care is still evolving and evaluations are needed. The engagement of professionals in evaluation of care is associated with the improvement of the quality of direct individualised care and stimulating personal and professional growth.

POST-READING EXERCISE 7.1 (ANSWERS ON PP. 109-10)

Time 40 minutes
1   What supportive conditions would you consider elementary for an Assertive Outreach Team in order to function properly?
    a.   From a professional team point of view

b. From an institutional point of view.
2 In what way can the Socratic conversation method contribute to professional development?
3 When reading about Liz, what would, in your opinion, be an efficient way to deal with the situation in order to accomplish a good transfer?

REFERENCES

1 Thompson KS, Griffith EE, Leaf PJ. A historical review of the Madison model of community care. *Hosp Community Psychiatry*. 1990; **41**: 625–34.

2 Wennink HJ, De Wilde GWMM, Van Weeghel J, *et al*. De metamorfose van de GGZ: kanttekeningen bij vermaatschappelijking. *MGv*. 2001; **56**: 917–37.

3 Stein LI, Test MA, editors. *Alternatives to Mental Hospital Treatment*. New York, NY, and London: Plenum Press; 1978.

4 Blok G. *Baas in eigen brein: 'Antipsychiatrie' in Nederland, 1965–1985*. Amsterdam: Uitgeverij Nieuwezijds; 2004.

5 Schene AH, Faber AME. Mental health care reform in the Netherlands. *Acta Psychiatr Scand*. 2001; **104**: 74–81 (s410).

6 Pijl YJ, Sytema S, Barels R, *et al*. Costs of deinstitutionalization in a rural catchment area in the Netherlands. *Psychol Med*. 2002; **32**: 1435–43.

7 McDaid D, Thornicroft G. *Policy Brief Mental Health II: balancing institutional and community-based care: World Health Organization, on behalf of the European Observatory on Health Systems and Policies*. 2005. Available at: www.euro.who.int/document/e85488.pdf (accessed 7 June 2010).

8 Test MA, Stein LI. Practical guidelines for the community treatment of markedly impaired patients. *Community Ment Health J*. 2000; **36**: 47–60.

9 Lachance KR, Santos AB. Modifying the PACT model: preserving critical elements. *Psychiatr Serv*. 1995; **46**: 601–4.

10 Wolf J, Mensink C, Van der Lubbe P, *et al*. *Casemanagement voor langdurig verslaafden met meervoudige problemen: een systematisch overzicht van interventie en effect*. Utrecht: Resultaten Scoren; 2002.

11 Intagliata J. Improving the quality of community care for the chronically mentally disabled: the role of case management. *Schizophr Bull*. 1982; **8**: 655–74.

12 Wingerson D, Ries RK. Assertive community treatment for patients with chronic and severe mental illness who abuse drugs. *J Psychoactive Drugs*. 1999; **31**: 13–18.

13 Rapp CA. The active ingredients of effective case management: a research synthesis. *Community Ment Health J*. 1998; **34**: 363–80.

14 Billings J, Johnson S, Bebbington P, *et al*. Assertive Outreach Teams in London: staff experiences and perceptions – Pan-London Assertive Outreach Study, Part 2. *Br J Psychiatry*. 2003; **183**: 139–47.

15 Mueser KT, Bond GR, Drake RE, *et al*. Models of community care for severe mental illness: a review of research on case management. *Schizophr Bull*. 1998; **24**: 37–74.

16 Henskens R. *Grab and hold: randomized controlled trial of the effectiveness of an outreach treatment program for chronic, high-risk crack abusers*. [doctoral dissertation]. Tilllburg: Tilburg University; 2004.

17 Bedell JR, Cohen NL, Sullivan A. Case management: the current best practices and the next generation of innovation. *Community Ment Health J*. 2000; **36**: 179–94.

18 Shepherd G. Case management. *Health Trends.* 1990; **22**: 59–61.

19 Burns T, Catty J. Assertive community treatment in the UK. *Psychiatr Serv.* 2002; **53**: 630–1.

20 Burns T, Creed F, Fahy T, *et al.* Intensive versus standard case management for severe psychotic illness: a randomised trial. *Lancet.* 1999; **353**: 2185–9.

21 Lohuis G, Schilperoort R, Schout G. *Van bemoei-naar groeizorg: Methodieken voor de OGGz.* Groningen: Wolters-Noordhoff bv; 2000.

22 Roeg DPK. *Measurement of program characteristics of intensive community-based care for persons with complex addiction problems* [doctoral dissertation]. Tillburg: Tilburg University; 2007. Available at: www.uvt.nl/tranzo/academischewerkplaatsen/vz/community basedcare.pdf (accessed 7 June 2010).

23 Van de Lindt S. *Bemoei je ermee: Leidraad voor assertieve psychiatrische hulp aan zorgmijders.* Assen: van Gorcum; 2000.

24 Young AS, Grusky O, Sullivan G, *et al.* The effect of provider characteristics on case management activities. *Adm Policy Ment Health.* 1998; **26**: 21–32.

25 Roeg DPK, van de Goor LAM, Garretsen HFL. Towards structural quality indicators for intensive community-based care programmes for substance abusers. *Community Ment Health J.* 2008; **44**: 405–15.

26 Roeg DPK, van de Goor LAM, Garretsen HFL. Towards quality indicators for assertive outreach programmes for severely impaired substance abusers: concept mapping with Dutch experts. *Int J Qual Health Care.* 2005; **17**: 203–8.

27 Hitchings KS, Davies-Hathen N, Capuano TA, *et al.* Peer case review sharpens event analysis. *J Nurs Care Qual.* 2008; **23**: 296–304.

28 Hargreaves WA, Jerrell JM, Lawless SF, *et al.* Doing the difficult and dangerous: the community program practice scale. *Admin Pol Ment Health.* 2007; **34**: 138–49.

29 Teague GB, Bond GR, Drake RE. Program fidelity in assertive community treatment: development and use of a measure. *Am J Orthopsychiatry.* 1998; **68**: 216–32.

30 Roeg DPK, van de Goor LAM, Garretsen HFL. Characterizing intensive community-based care: use, reliability and factor structure of a generic measure. *Ment Health Subst Use.* 2008; **1**: 158–71.

31 Hall M, Meaden A, Smith J, *et al.* Brief report: the development and psychometric properties of an observer-rated measure of engagement with mental health services. *J Ment Health.* 2001; **10**: 457–65.

32 Wing JK, Beevor AS, Curtis RH, *et al.* Health of the Nation Outcome Scales (HoNOS); research and development. *Br J Psychiatry.* 1998; **172**: 11–18.

33 Kennedy JA. *Mastering the Kennedy Axis V: a new psychiatric assessment of patient functioning.* Washington, DC: American Psychiatric Publishing; 2003.

34 Priebe S, Huxley P, Knight S, Evans S. Application and results of the Manchester Short Assessment of Quality of Life (Mansa). *Int J Soc Psychiatry.* 1999; **45**: 7–12.

35 Schon D. *The Reflective Practitioner: how professionals think in action.* London: Temple Smith; 1983.

EXERCISE ANSWERS

ANSWERS TO PRE-READING EXERCISE 7.1

1 Community-based care is an alternative for the psychiatric hospital and is aimed at persons with severe mental health–substance use problems. Services are provided in the person's own environment and training is available to aid community living. Intensive variants are characterised by an outgoing approach of service providers, high frequent contact, and care coordination. It is aimed at persons with complex and combined problems that, by themselves, do not reach healthcare and/or cannot find their way in the fragmentised healthcare system. Examples are:

   - training in community living
   - assertive community treatment
   - Assertive Outreach Teams
   - Community Mental Health Teams
   - interferential care
   - case management.

2 About 50 years ago, the mental healthcare system changed dramatically. Under the influence of anti-psychiatry, many psychiatric hospitals closed their wards. Different ambulant services came into existence. They were aimed at previously hospitalised persons with severe mental health and or substance use (alcohol and drugs – prescribed and illicit) problems. The aim was to support persons to live in society. The living circumstances for most people improved enormously. However, for some 'living in the community' appeared too much and too soon. It was for them that intensive variants of community-based care came into existence.

ANSWERS TO POST-READING EXERCISE 7.1

1a For a professional team it is important that community-based methods are considered effective. Every professional should show a positive and constructive attitude towards the applied techniques in general. At the same time, professionals should encourage the use of a personal style. An open mind is required to reflect on care issues characterised by moral dimensions. A team leader who is not biased (e.g. cooperation of different organisations), who can enforce team spirit by celebrating small successes, can prevent exposure to unnecessary stress and frustration. The professional should have a balanced caseload and should experience shared team responsibility.

1b Healthcare organisations should become more sensitive to methods of community based care. Acknowledgement of structural facilities to respond to the needs of a individual can be understood as a fundamental condition for the continuation of community based care. Moreover, it is a crucial condition to support the professional that wants to 'survive' in the long term.

2 The Socratic conversation method invites the professional (unqualified and qualified) to reflect thoroughly on a care issue in which they are involved. Moreover, this offers an opportunity to discuss personal convictions about basic human understanding; the provisional character of judgement; and enables professional insight in motives of a concrete approach. This can result in better justification of the applied techniques and approach. In general, effective methods of team reflection can contribute to a sense of shared responsibility and solid position within an organisation.

3 When a professional is confronted with a collegial disagreement on the terms for transfer of an individual, and for care continuation, there are several options:
- The cause for the collegial disagreement could be found in former treatment episodes that might have been problematic. It is important to discuss the actual goals and opportunity that lies ahead for the individual. Colleges can have legitimate objections to agree with the actual terms, due to a cumbersome past relationship. To create new opportunities in a professional and objective care relation, a different care continuator may be required:
- When underlying method of intensive community-based care is not understood by supportive health organisation, clear communication is needed via appropriate management channels to change mindset. A professional must be aware of the organisational conditions that facilitate community-based methods. A team leader or psychiatrist can indicate that there is a lack of structural support and plead for managers to take responsibility, setting proper directives.

CHAPTER 8

Guidelines for working with mental health–substance use

Elizabeth Hughes

INTRODUCTION

This chapter addresses clinical guidelines and their purpose, with an emphasis on how they may apply to people with mental health–substance use problems. Examples of specific international clinical guidelines will be examined. The chapter concludes with some recommendations and discussion.

WHAT ARE CLINICAL GUIDELINES?

The National Institute for Health and Clinical Excellence (NICE) in England define clinical guidelines as

> *recommendations on the appropriate treatment and care of people with specific diseases and conditions . . .* [and] *are based on the best available evidence.*[1]

Guidelines are developed to target a specific health problem, and have a number of purposes:

➤ to provide recommendations for treatment and care of people by professionals
➤ to develop standards of care (which can be audited and evaluated)
➤ as part of education and training of professionals
➤ to assist people in making informed choices about the type of treatment they receive and improve communication between persons receiving care and professionals providing care.

However, guidelines only provide *guidance* on practice, and each professional is accountable for their interpretation and implementation of the guidelines for each individual to whom they offer intervention and treatment. Therefore, it is important that a person is treated as a unique individual. Sometimes the complex health and social situation may require the professional (unqualified and qualified) to deviate from the guidance to offer best care. For people with mental health–substance use problems this is particularly pertinent. It is likely that each person who falls into this group will have treatment needs that cut across several clinical guidelines.

Scenario: Ruth

> Ruth, 25, has a 9-year history of heroin use, and is currently on a slow reduction methadone programme. Ruth has recently discovered that she is hepatitis C positive and is receiving treatment for this from a liver specialist. Ruth has also experienced depression and anxiety for several years, and is seeing a primary care counselor for this. Ruth is 4 months pregnant and is receiving care from a specialist substance use antenatal clinic.

Q: CONSIDER – HOW MANY CLINICAL GUIDELINES MIGHT RUTH'S TREATMENT COVER?

 TIME OUT: Take 5 minutes to reflect on this question. Make notes of your conclusions before reading on.

Ruth's treatment will cross at least four clinical guidelines for:
1 methadone prescribing
2 treatment of hepatitis C
3 psychosocial interventions for depression and anxiety
4 pregnancy.

However, treatment for one condition may adversely affect another – for example, Ribavirin (medication for the treatment of hepatitis) is contraindicated in pregnancy.

CLINICAL GUIDELINES FOR MENTAL HEALTH–SUBSTANCE USE

As demonstrated, some of the difficulties in providing treatment for people with mental health–substance use is that they invariably require treatment for a range of problems (sometimes from different types of services) at the same time. This may include psychosocial and medical interventions. This means their treatment will fall under different clinical guidelines at the same time. There are often tensions between the two sets of guidelines, which can, at the very least, cause confusion for the individual – by receiving conflicting information and approaches – and at worst, receive treatment that has dangerous interactions with a concurrent treatment from another service. Due to the complicated interplay of mental health and substance use, treatment decisions may have to contradict clinical guidelines for one of the problems. This means that multi-agency, and professional communication is vital regarding all aspects of treatment, and lead professionals should coordinate. In England, the Care Coordinator under the Care Programme Approach,[2] may take responsibility.

KEY POINT 8.1

It is very important that all professionals prescribing medication to a person are communicating about the prescribing practices to ensure that there are no drug interactions or adverse effects.

Scenario: Joe

Joe, 40, has a long history of psychotic illness. He had been under the local mental health team for many years, and at least once a year, became so unwell that he required hospitalisation due to paranoid delusions and suicidal thoughts. In addition, Joe was a heavy drinker (he came from a family of heavy drinkers). Joe's drinking affected his mental state in several ways including lowering his mood and forgetting to take his medication. He was prescribed Olanzapine by the psychiatrist, and the community nurse monitored his prescribed dose. Joe was referred to the local substance use (drug and alcohol) team. Joe was assessed regarding his chaotic drinking. In light of his limited motivation and previous difficulty abstaining, he was prescribed Disulfiram by the substance use team psychiatrist.

Q: CONSIDER – WHAT OBSERVATIONS HAVE YOU MADE? WHAT WOULD BE YOUR CONCLUSIONS?

 TIME OUT: Take 5 minutes to reflect on this question. Make notes of your conclusions before reading on.

Disulfiram is contraindicated for people with psychosis as it can exacerbate it, but in Joe's case the risk of him drinking and becoming severely paranoid and suicidal was more significant than the risk of Disulfiram exacerbating his illness. This decision was discussed and shared between the team and Joe at a Care Programme Approach care review.

There are significant challenges in the development of coherent guidelines for people experiencing mental health–substance use problems. Any clinical guidelines developed need to balance a fine line, taking into account the latest evidence-based practice, while trying to avoid being too prescriptive and rigid.

KEY POINT 8.2

Service provision needs to be individualised and flexible, while maintaining quality standards and consistency.

THE USA

Integrated services for mental health–substance use have been developed, and evaluated in the USA since the late 1980s. The most prolific developments have occurred in New Hampshire.[3] Minkoff[4] developed a set of clinical guidelines for mental health–substance use, which are based on the developments in integrated treatment in the USA. The principles of this model have heavily influenced the development of guidance across the world. Therefore, it is important to focus on this first.

The first section of the guidelines outlines seven principals of the Integrated Treatment Model.

1 Co-occurring mental health and substance use problems are normal, not an exception. Therefore, all services (mental health and substance use) should be ready and able to work the individual experiencing mental health–substance use problems.

2 Organised into four sub-groups (*see* Figure 2.1 on p. 18)[5] depending on severity of the mental health and substance use issues.

3 Treatment outcomes are enhanced by integrating interventions from mental health and substance use continuously. Progress is usually incremental, and evidence suggests no one type of intervention is more effective. Therefore, a range of interventions should be available, and tailored to the individual.

4 Integrated dual primary diagnosis specific interventions – should apply the appropriate evidence-based treatments for each separate disorder such as psychopharmacology, trauma therapy.

5 Interventions should be matched to stage of recovery and level of motivation to make certain changes.

6 There is no single dual disorders set of interventions; there should be a range of interventions available so that the treatment can be tailor-made to an individual's specific needs, and choices.

7 Outcomes should be individualised and not just based on abstinence, but on a whole range of levels of use, methods of use, reduction in psychiatric symptoms, stage of change, use of services and reduction of harm.[4]

The guidance moves on to defining the group that this is aimed at:

> *Any psychiatric disorder (including both Axis I and Axis II disorders, as well as substance-induced psychiatric disorders), combined with substance dependence and/or abuse. N.B. For individuals with Severe Mental Illness associated with persistent disability, any persistent pattern of substance use may be defined as abuse.*[4 p. 4]

Practice standards

As mental health–substance use problems are expected, and the norm, all services should offer a welcoming, and engaging reception to all individuals experiencing mental health–substance use problems, no matter what the issues may be. Assessment should start at this point, and there should be no expectation on the person for them to self-define as having a 'mental health' and/or 'substance use problem'. There should be no barriers to accessing mental health or substance use services based on having other co-occurring problems. People should be able to access continuity of care through a specific person or team over the long term. There needs to be a delicate balance struck between giving care, but also empowering the individual to take responsibility – when able – and control over their lives and choices. The professional should empathically confront the person with some of the negative consequences of their lifestyle choices. Each problem should receive the appropriate treatment. Treatment should be structured in stages according to the level of engagement and motivation of the person:

➤ active stabilisation
➤ motivational enhancement
➤ active treatment
➤ relapse prevention
➤ rehabilitation and recovery.

As well as appropriate treatment, other important areas of rehabilitation and recovery need to be addressed including:

➤ housing
➤ social contacts
➤ employment
➤ meaningful activity.

Treatment should be coordinated and collaborative, and should include the families, carers, and other agencies/professionals.

Assessment

Assessment is an ongoing process, it should be carefully structured and take place over a period of time. Initial assessment and diagnosis should be treated as presumptive, and subject to continual re-evaluation. Screening tools for substance use and mental health should be used in mental health and substance use settings (*see* To learn more). Where a mental health and substance use problem(s) co-exist, even if the mental health problems is thought to be substance use-induced, both should be considered primary and receive the appropriate treatment. Attention should be paid in assessment to common mental health–substance use issues, such as:

➤ history of trauma
➤ cognitive impairment
➤ personality traits, and disorders
➤ other health issues – sexually transmitted diseases, blood-borne viruses
➤ other health conditions associated with mental health and or substance use problems.

Assessment of strengths, and levels of impairment are also very important in ensuring that the level of support provided is individualised.

Treatment

Where treatment is provided will depend on the sub-group category of mental health–substance use the person best fits (*see* Chapter 2, Figure 2.1, p. 18).[5] If the substance use is the most severe problem, then substance use services should be providing integrated care; if the mental health issue is severe, then mental health should be providing this. A range of services, according to individual needs, should provide treatment. This can include:

➤ case management teams
➤ assertive outreach
➤ Crisis Teams
➤ supported housing
➤ inpatient facilities.

Across the whole spectrum of mental health and substance use services. External contingencies can also be used, and these include:

➤ payee-ships
➤ abstinence-expected housing
➤ conditions of probation.

There are many laudable qualities in the Minkoff guidelines,[4] many of these principles have been adopted internationally. However, in terms of cultural context, it is important to mention the tensions that do exist in the USA around substance use treatment. Many states in the USA do not offer methadone programmes, needle exchanges, or other harm-minimisation approaches. A mainly abstinence approach is adopted in many places. Given this as a context, makes the person-centred approach of the New Hampshire model highly unusual. This type of integrated treatment is not the norm across the USA. In addition, the mental health services have more powers of compulsion over treatment adherence than perhaps in other countries. People released from county hospitals on a licence can be recalled instantly if they breech the conditions of their release. This may include non-adherence to medication, and not attending group therapy for example. However, this also means that people are less likely to slip through the net, and relapse of both mental health and substance use are picked up rapidly, and dealt with.

ENGLAND

In 2002, the Department of Health published a good practice guide for people with serious mental health problems and additional substance use problems.[6] The evidence base for the guidance was heavily based on research conducted in the USA (focusing on Drake *et al.*[3] work). This guide was aimed specifically at those people already in the secondary mental health services, i.e. those with severe mental health–substance use problems.

The guidance set out clearly for the first time the direction of travel for mental health/substance use treatment in England. The concept of 'mainstreaming' was introduced, and adopted Minkoff's[4] premise that substance use was usual rather than exceptional in people experiencing mental health problems. Unlike the New Hampshire model of integrated treatment teams, the vision was to educate and train professionals in mental health (primarily) to work with substance use issues in an 'integrated' fashion. Integration in England refers to the use of therapeutic approaches that are an amalgamation and modification of approaches used separately for mental health and substance use. It also includes adherence to the principles of Integrated Treatment model of New Hampshire:

➤ longitudinal approach
➤ flexible
➤ setting small goals
➤ collaborative
➤ assertive engagement
➤ stage-wise approach
➤ working with the wider circle of peers and families/carers.

All local areas were to develop their own strategy for working with people experiencing mental health–substance use problems, and should include multi-agency/professional approach and collaboration; including third-sector organisations, as well as statutory. The *Good Practice Guide*[6] did not make specific clinical recommendations about the treatment of people with mental health–substance use.

In 2006, the Department of Health published guidance on working with substance use issues in mental health inpatient and day hospital facilities.[7] This document aimed to set out clear guidance to tackle the very specific issues of substance use while a person has an admission for a mental health problem. This guidance was focused on the clinical management of specific issues including:

➤ assessment
➤ obtaining and testing samples for drug testing (such as, urine screening)
➤ setting realistic substance-related goals
➤ working with other agencies/professionals, family and carers
➤ management of substance use-related incidents on the ward (e.g. dealing, intoxication).

In 2007, the updated clinical guidelines for drug dependence were published (known as the 'Orange Guidelines').[8] This sets out clear and evidence-based guidance for the effective treatment of drug dependency (mainly focused on opiate dependency) including assessment, prescribing and detoxification. Within the Orange Guidelines, there is a section specifically for people with additional mental health problems, as well as drug dependency. It is acknowledged that people with drug dependency may also have mental health problems, and that they require high quality, person-focused integrated care with mental health services. People with sufficient levels of risk or severity of mental health problems should be under the Care Programme Approach,[2] usually led by mental health services. However, local arrangements may mean that substance use service may care coordinate. Because of the high prevalence of mental health problems, substance use services should ensure that all people using the service receive a comprehensive assessment that includes their mental health needs, and ensures that where these needs are identified steps are taken to address them working jointly and flexibly with mental health services

WALES

In Wales, a service framework was developed to meet the needs of people with mental health and substance use problems.[9] Not specifically guidelines for clinical management, but Appendix A has a good practice checklist that sets out minimum expectations for service delivery.

SCOTLAND

In Scotland their guidance, Mind the Gaps,[10] had more of a service development focus than specific clinical guidance, and recommends a diverse skills mix to address needs, including confident professionals to delivering interventions, and generic professionals competent to deal with the less complex issues in partnership with substance use services. They take a focus on the importance of good assessment to obtain a complete picture of all their health and social needs. Interventions recommended are based on integrated treatment:

➤ engagement
➤ attending to basic needs
➤ persuasion
➤ active intervention
➤ early intervention.

AUSTRALIA

In Australia, each state is responsible for developing their own health policy and guidelines. New South Wales has recently published a new version of clinical guidelines for people with mental health–substance use problems.[11]

Comorbidity is defined as:

> Situations where people have problems related both to their use of substances (from hazardous through to harmful use and/or dependence) and to their mental health (from problematic symptoms through to highly prevalent conditions, such as, depression and anxiety, to the low prevalence disorders such as psychosis) (p. 7).[11]

The guidelines scope provides professionals with information to guide care, but it is not intended to replace expert clinical opinion. They adopt a philosophy of 'no wrong door':

> This 'no wrong door' principle clarifies that the responsibility of providing care that addresses the range of client needs is the responsibility of the care provider/service where the client presents ... This requires services to provide care, and/or facilitate access to service delivery that falls beyond their specific focus. It removes the onus of negotiating different services and providers from the client and thereby aims to reduce the incidence of clients 'falling through the cracks' of a complex service delivery system (p. 6).[11]

Thus, responsibility lies with all services. No one service can opt out of providing care for people experiencing mental health–substance use problems. The guidelines covers treatment issues, such as engaging people into treatment, service delineations using a variation on Minkoff's[4] quadrant. It defines integrated treatment as

> the provision of mental health and substance use treatment by one clinician or within one service where the clinicians assume responsibility for synthesising information and ensuring that a client moves toward recovery with a consistent approach and consistent information (p. 18).[11]

This takes many forms, from separate and specialist mental health–substance use services, or where general services adapt providing integrated, as a routine, care. In addition, it describes parallel and sequential care, but advises that these latter models are not effective and should be avoided. The components of treatment are then presented in more detail starting with screening, assessment, management of acute crisis and withdrawal from substances. Many of the components and philosophy mirrors that of Minkoff,[4] but with the additional focus on harm reduction and diversity that is limited in the Minkoff guidelines.[4] Assessment should be comprehensive and long term, and involve an exploration of all aspects of a person's life and functioning. It emphasises the importance of risk assessment and focuses particularly on suicide risk. A further section gives an overview of mental health problems including anxiety, mood, psychosis and personality disorders, the likely presentations of these, treatments, interactions between mental health and substance use problems, and medications, and further resources relevant to these issues. There is a section on specific populations within this group relevant to the geographical area including:
➤ young people
➤ the person with hepatitis C or HIV
➤ rural and remote people
➤ homeless
➤ indigenous populations
➤ gay, lesbian
➤ bi-sexual
➤ transgender
➤ older adults
➤ people with chronic pain
➤ people from diverse ethnic groups.

The NSW guidelines[11] are very comprehensive and well resourced. However, there are a few gaps. There is mention of risk of violence and offending, running through the guidelines, but it specifically only focuses on suicide risk. There are also many other serious risks associated with mental health–substance use, such as:
➤ violence towards others or property
➤ victimisation and abuse
➤ health risks – accidental overdose and blood-borne viruses, and self-neglect.

Risk assessment and management should be more comprehensive and include the whole range of risk outcomes. In addition, the NSW guidelines[11] focus on the main mental health issues, but does not include a similar section on substance use issues.

DISCUSSION

Guidelines are only good and useful if they are implemented. So many policy and clinical guidelines are published, but how far do they get implemented? In the UK, the Themed Review for Mental Health,[8] focused on assessing how far the recommendations from the *Dual Diagnosis Good Practice Guide*,[6] had been implemented across local areas. The outcome was that implementation was extremely patchy. Some regions of the country had strategies, training programmes, and specific services and pathways developed for people with mental health–substance use; whereas some areas had not even managed to achieve a local agreement on definition of mental health–substance use. The National Dual Diagnosis Programme,[12] has developed a number of products including training resources, a carers DVD and documents regarding developing capable professionals and capable strategies. These resources have gone some way in developing and implementing the recommendations from the *Good Practice Guide*.[6]

RECOMMENDATIONS
Local champions

The key to implementation of clinical guidelines are the people in the local areas including people using the service, family, carers and professionals. Where implementation has worked, is where senior local leads drive forward change within services and within practice.

Access to knowledge

In order to implement guidelines, people need access to such documents. Many guidelines are now accessible via the Internet, and it is important that people are aware of these guidelines and gain access to these documents. Guidelines may need to be written in two forms:
1 for the layperson
2 for the professionally qualified – to address the varying needs of the individual in terms of level of information.

In addition, some attention should be paid to whether the guidelines are available in other languages, or in formats suitable for those with visual impairments. Local champions/leads should play a central role in the dissemination of clinical guidelines to all stakeholders.

Education and training

All professionals (unqualified and qualified) employed to work with people and their families in relation to mental health–substance use, should have access to evidence-based education and training. The content should be allied to the local and national guidelines and include local knowledge regarding patterns of substance use, service configuration and local strategies. People accessing the service, the family and carers should be involved in the development, delivery and evaluation of such education and training initiatives.

Practice development and supervision

All professionals working with people experiencing mental health–substance use problems should, as a matter of course, receive good quality ongoing supervision from a suitably experienced and knowledgeable professional regarding clinical guidance, interventions and treatment. This ensures that competence developed through education, training and clinical practice, is enhanced, and developed through reflective practice and continued learning opportunities.

KEY POINT 8.3

Supervision ensures safe and effective practice in line with appropriate clinical guidance.

CONCLUSION

Clinical guidelines are only as good as the people implementing them. Many documents describe best practice for mental health–substance use. However, we need to make it our business to ensure that we:

➤ are aware of the local and national clinical guidelines
➤ understand the complexities of providing treatment for people experiencing multiple needs
➤ are committed to providing an equitable, safe, evidence- and values-based quality care for one of the most vulnerable groups of individuals currently using services.

REFERENCES

1 National Institute for Health and Clinical Excellence (NICE) *Clinical Guidelines*. 2010. Available at: http://www.guidance.nice.org.uk/CG (accessed 7 June 2010).
2 Department of Health. *Refocusing the Care Programme Approach: policy and positive practice guidance*. 2008. Available at: www.dh.gov.uk/prod_consum_dh/groups/dh_digitalassets/@dh/@en/documents/digitalasset/dh_083649.pdf (accessed 7 June 2010).
3 Drake RE, Gregory J, McHugo GJ, *et al.* Ten-year recovery outcomes for clients with co-occurring schizophrenia and substance use disorders. *Schizophr Bull.* 2006; **32**: 464–73.
4 Minkoff K. *Service Planning Guidelines Co-occurring Psychiatric And Substance Use Disorders.* 2001. Available at: www.bhrm.org/guidelines/Minkoff.pdf (accessed 7 June 2010).
5 NASMHPD/NASADAD. *National Dialogue on Co-Occurring Mental Health and Substance Abuse Disorders.* Washington, DC: NASMHPD; 1998. Available at: www.nasmhpd.org general_files/publications/NASADAD%20NASMHPD%20PUBS/National%20Dialogue pdf (accessed 7 June 2010).
6 Department of Health. *Mental Health Policy Implementation Guide: dual diagnosis good practice guide.* London: Department of Health; 2002. Available at: www.dh.gov.uk

prod_consum_dh/groups/dh_digitalassets/@dh/@en/documents/digitalasset/dh_4060435. pdf (accessed 7 June 2010).

7 Department of Health. *Dual Diagnosis Guidance for Psychiatric Inpatient and Day Hospital Facilities.* 2006. Available at: www.dh.gov.uk/prod_consum_dh/groups/dh_digitalassets/@ dh/@en/documents/digitalasset/dh_062652.pdf (accessed 7 June 2010).

8 Department of Health. *Themed Review Report 07: dual diagnosis. Executive summary.* 2007. Available at: www.nmhdu.org.uk/silo/files/dual-diagosis-themed-review-executive-summary-2007.pdf (accessed 7 June 2010).

9 Welsh Assembly Government. *A Service Framework to Meet the Needs of People with a Co-occurring Substance Misuse and Mental Health Problem.* 2007. Available at: www.wales. gov.uk/docs/dsjlg/publications/commsafety/090722cooccurringen.pdf (accessed 7 June 2010).

10 Scottish Advisory Committee on Drug Misuse (SACDM) and Scottish Advisory Committee on Alcohol Misuse (SACAM). *MIND THE GAPS: Meeting the needs of people with co-occurring substance misuse and mental health problems. Report of the joint working group.* 2003. Available at: www.scotland.gov.uk/Publications/2003/10/18358/28079 (accessed 7 June 2010).

11 New South Wales Department of Health. *New South Wales Clinical Guidelines for the Care of Persons with Comorbid Mental Illness and Substance Use Disorders in Acute Care Settings.* Sydney, NSW: New South Wales Department of Health; 2009. Available at: www.health.nsw. gov.au/pubs/2009/pdf/comorbidity_report.pdf (accessed 7 June 2010).

12 Department of Health. *New Horizons: a shared vision for mental health.* 2009. Available at: www.newhorizons.dh.gov.uk/assets/2010–02–04–299060_NewHorizons_acc2.pdf (accessed 7 June 2010).

TO LEARN MORE

- National Mental Health Development Unit: www.nmhdu.org.uk
- Alcohol Improvement Programme screening and assessment tools: www.alcohollearning centre.org.uk/Topics/Browse/BriefAdvice/
- National Institute on Alcohol Abuse and Alcoholism (USA) Screening for Alcohol Use and Alcohol Related Problems: http://pubs.niaaa.nih.gov/publications/aa65/aa65.htm

CHAPTER 9

Strategy development, model policy and procedures

Amanda J Barrett

PRE-READING EXERCISE 9.1

Before reading this chapter, consider the following questions, then review your reflections after reading this chapter:
- How does strategy differ from policy?
- What drivers exist locally to highlight the need for change in provision for meeting the needs of individuals experiencing mental health–substance use problems?
- What steps are required to devise and implement strategy and policy regarding the care of these individuals?
- What main issues need to be included in a policy to clarify arrangements for service provision?
- What needs to be included in a policy for training and developing professionals?

INTRODUCTION

Providing care for individuals with mental health and substance use needs reveals challenges and dilemmas in bringing about systemic change in complex organisations. Wide-ranging attitudes and beliefs about the person experiencing mental health–substance use problems means they may experience a variety of responses when trying to access services. To minimise such variation, it is vital that organisations standardise how services and professionals (unqualified and qualified) react to individuals experiencing mental health–substance use (drugs – legal/illegal and alcohol) needs. An essential part of the process of standardising care and promoting consistency is the development of strategy, policy and procedure to outline how professionals, services, organisations, and healthcare systems are required to respond.

A strategy is required to provide a clear statement of intent and specific objectives regarding plans for developing services for those experiencing mental health–substance use needs.

DRIVERS
National drivers

A number of policy and guidance documents have been published to steer the process of devising organisational systems, and developing professionals, that are capable of working with concurrent needs.

Prevalence studies

National prevalence data suggests that needs and presentation of individuals has changed,[1] with over 85% of people using alcohol services experiencing mental health problems, and 44% of people using mental health service found to be using substances.

National Service Framework

The National Service Framework (England) was developed in 1999,[2] setting out arrangements for planning, delivery and monitoring of services. For the individual experiencing mental health–substance use needs, the Framework states that care should be provided from within existing mental health and substance use services.

Dual Diagnosis Good Practice Guide

Published in 2002, the *Good Practice Guide* (England),[3] outlines the main considerations for developing effective services and their implementation to move towards integrated provision in mainstream mental health services. However, no specific targets, timescales, outcome indicators, or funding were attached to this guidance. Consequently, implementation has been patchy. An *Autumn Assessment Themed Review* (England),[4] was conducted in 2007, to determine what progress had been made in implementing the *Good Practice Guide*. At the time of the review, only 60% of Local Implementation Teams had a locally agreed mental health–substance use strategy.

Closing the Gap: capability framework

In collaboration with the Care Services Improvement Partnership, the Centre for Clinical and Academic Workforce Innovation developed a capability framework,[5] to assist organisations in appraising and developing professional capability in working effectively with mental health–substance use problems. The framework is aimed at all organisations working with individual experiencing mental health–substance use problems, with 19 capabilities derived from a number of capability and competency-based frameworks relevant to the fields of mental health and substance use. The capabilities are intended to be achieved at three possible levels (core, generalist or specialist) depending upon the requirements of professional roles.

Mental health inpatient and day hospital guidance

In 2006, the Department of Health produced guidance for National Health Service, social services, voluntary and private sector organisations on the assessment and management of people with mental illness who also use substances in mental health hospital settings.[6] The guide clearly states that assessment and management of the care are core competencies of mental health professionals.

Dual Diagnosis Good Practice Handbook

The *Good Practice Handbook* was developed by Turning Point,[7] to build upon existing guidance by demonstrating how it has been successfully implemented across a range of treatment settings and providers in England. The handbook facilitates sharing of good practice, through the use of case studies, and encourages professionals and service providers to get in touch to exchange information.

National Service Framework: five years on

In reviewing progress in implementing the National Service Framework, the Department of Health,[8] highlighted that meeting the needs of those with mental health–substance use needs is *'one of the most pressing problems facing mental health services today'.* The review stresses the importance of a broad coordinated response from services based on collaboration between services, professional training, and prevention of substance use.

Clinical Negligence Scheme for Trusts

The National Health Service Litigation Authority (NHSLA) developed the Clinical Negligence Scheme for Trusts,[9] a voluntary scheme for improving service standards relating to risks. Foundation Trusts are required to achieve level one as a minimum. In 2008, NHSLA introduced additional standards relating to mental health–substance use, setting out requirements for service providers in three levels.

1 **Level 1**: requires that documentation be agreed within the organisation (e.g. a policy) setting out arrangements for the individual experiencing mental health–substance misuse needs.
2 **Level 2**: requires evidence to demonstrate that the policy has been implemented.
3 **Level 3**: requires evidence that recommendations and action plans have been developed and implemented to overcome any gaps or deficits identified during the monitoring process.

Refocusing the Care Programme Approach

A review of the Care Programme Approach,[10] has been carried out to ensure consistency and reduce bureaucracy in planning, organising and delivering care. The review includes specific reference to the care of individuals experiencing mental health–substance use needs, highlighting that all assessments in mental health services should include:

➤ consideration of substance use
➤ assessment of risk
➤ risk management planning.

Developing a capable dual diagnosis strategy

A new guidance document[11] outlined key steps and considerations for commissioners and lead providers of services in developing local mental health–substance use strategies.

Local drivers

Although policies and guidance documents exist at national level, they only become meaningful when applied to the local situation.

Findings of needs assessment

Assessing need will highlight local gaps, barriers and enablers relating to care provision. It is a critical part of the process as locally relevant, meaningful strategy and policy will flow from this essential piece of work.

DEVELOPING STRATEGY

The Department of Health *Dual Diagnosis Good Practice Guide*,[3] provides a useful insight into the process of developing dual diagnosis strategy.

Establish the project team

Establishing the project team is vital as it provides leadership and impetus for development and implementation of the strategy. The *Dual Diagnosis Good Practice Guide*,[3] sets out arrangements for establishing and running a project team, ensuring that the right organisations are represented by professionals who are in a position to influence and make necessary decisions within their own organisations (*see* Box 9.1). Creating a project team ensures drive from commissioners, permitting financial and strategic collaboration between organisations.

BOX 9.1 Project team composition

- Lead commissioner.
- Provider manager.
- Clinical representatives from mental health and substance use.
- One of the above to be a lead clinician.
- Local Implementation Team representative.
- Drug Action Team representative.
- Administrative support.

Agreeing the scope

Once the project team is assembled, it is important to agree the scope of the strategy to ensure that groups or services are not excluded. Representation on the project team will strongly influence the scope of the strategy. A strategy with a broad scope will increase the opportunity for inclusion of people with a range of needs and involve a wider range of providers. A broad scope will also generate a more extensive implementation plan and require greater commitment of resources (*see* Box 9.2).

Engaging stakeholders

Engaging core and interested stakeholders is a key stage in the process in order to ensure their ownership, and involvement in the process. This is critical to ensure that the strategy addresses their concerns and sets realistic, achievable goals.

BOX 9.2 Possible considerations to discuss when agreeing the strategy scope

- Will the strategy include primary and secondary care, statutory and non-statutory providers?
- Does the strategy relate to a specific age or group of individuals?
- Is the strategy limited by specific geographical locations or organisational boundaries?
- How are the stakeholders organisations reached and consulted during the process?

Stakeholder involvement needs to occur throughout the process of developing and implementing strategy, and services. This can be achieved in many different ways. The most effective methods are based on the needs of each stakeholder 'audience', and revolve around existing structures within stakeholder groups, such as regular meetings with individuals using the services.

Agreeing definitions

Agreeing a definition that works within the whole system of mental health and substance use service provision requires a broad scope that includes a range of individuals experiencing varying degrees of severity and complexity of needs. The definition dictates the service model and policy changes to follow, a broad definition minimises the risk of individuals being excluded from services. Focusing on need, rather than diagnosis facilitates this, as people experiencing mental health–substance use problems who have experienced difficulty accessing services often do not reach the point of being formally diagnosed before dropping out of services. The complexity of the process and time required to develop the locally agreed definition of mental health–substance use must not be underestimated. Differing viewpoints of the various stakeholder organisations can complicate the process, as they are mindful of their own service specifications and eligibility criteria. Stakeholders may find it difficult to reconcile the strategic view of the wider care system with their own service perspective. The agreed definition directly affects the model of service delivery chosen (*see* Box 9.3). A broad definition that includes a range of mental health and substance use needs will give higher rates of prevalence when conducting needs assessment. In areas where the majority of people present with mental health–substance use needs it is not viable to develop an additional service to deal specifically with these people.

Needs assessment

Identifying the local position is crucial to effectively devising a strategy to apply national policy and guidance. Analysing local need is a vital step to establish:
- local prevalence
- individual, family and carer experiences
- barriers to services
- current provision
- professional capabilities and attitudes.

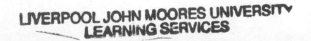

BOX 9.3 Key issues to consider when agreeing a definition

- The scope of the strategy agreed with commissioners and stakeholders will affect the specific details of the definition.
- Are individual with a range of mental health and substance use needs included or does the definition focus on more severe cases?
- Local needs assessment will be based on this definition and therefore will impact on prevalence data.
- Are individual using the service defined by their formal diagnosis or presenting needs?
- How will stakeholders be consulted on devising the definition?
- The process may be lengthy and involve considerable debate.

This will identify local gaps and provide the baseline for developments. The *Dual Diagnosis Good Practice Guide*,[3] offers a useful starting point to the process of assessing needs by suggesting some questions to ask local stakeholders and advocates avoiding carrying out lengthy local prevalence studies. It is important to get an approximate view of perceived local need and prevalence of mental health–substance use need, including local levels of severity, substances used and presenting mental health needs. The needs assessment will also identify individual, family, carer and professional views regarding gaps and barriers to accessing and providing effective services. Local knowledge regarding organisational structures and processes can be invaluable, as local meetings and events can be used during the needs assessment to reach stakeholders, without the lengthy process of organising special events to reach them. During the needs assessment process, individuals may emerge who have the attitude and capabilities to be local leaders; valuable assets to planning, and implementing strategy and policy.

Local service plan
The project team devises a local service plan to address the issues identified by the needs assessment. This will form the basis of the strategy to follow.

Service model
Agreeing the service model is crucial to the process of devising the local service plan as it clarifies how services will work together in delivering care. While there is limited evidence that a particular model is effective in providing care for the person experiencing mental health–substance use problems, guidance points us towards using an integrated model,[3] whereby care is provided from a single service. A collaborative approach, where mental health and substance use services work closely to deliver care from a single care plan, can be used as an interim step towards an integrated approach. This is due to the need to develop capability and confidence in professionals working with the individual experiencing mental health–substance use needs, as collaborative care provision between services enables professionals to gain experience and development opportunities, while ensuring that individuals receive the care and expertise deserved. Professionals experience and capability

must be explored during the needs assessment and considered when agreeing the service provision model to ensure that a gap does not exist between professionals roles and capabilities. Setting out consistent referral and care pathways is important to clarify how services operate collaboratively within the wider system of care provision and reassures professionals that their roles and caseloads are clearly defined.

Draft strategy

Members of the project team will develop and agree a draft version of the strategy. It simplifies the process if one professional leads in drafting and circulating the document, rather than hold a lengthy series of meetings to write the strategy.

Consultation process

A plan is required to establish how stakeholders will be reached during the consultation phase and identify who is responsible for circulating the draft and collating feedback. Consulting widely and thoroughly is essential to ensure that stakeholders are involved and engaged in the process and that the strategy addresses relevant issues and concerns.

Finalise and ratify

Comments received from the consultation phase are discussed. Then the project team produces a final draft strategy. Executive-level professionals in the stakeholder organisations – to ensure that it is fully supported and disseminated in the implementation stage – must then ratify the strategy.

POLICY DEVELOPMENT

Why are policies required?

If a strategy is a statement of purpose and long-term objectives achieve this, a policy can be thought of as current systems and processes in place to implement goals and objectives within an organisation.[1] Devising and implementing formal policies and procedures based upon strategic goals is an integral part of making this happen. This is due to professionals within an organisation being charged with implementing its policies and procedures, as stated in the job description and contract of employment. Other organisational policies will need to be reviewed to reflect the care required including:

➤ training policies
➤ professional (unqualified and qualified) development
➤ Care Programme Approach.

Policy components

The main components of a comprehensive policy outlining the care of those with mental health–substance use needs should include the following five components:

Scope of the policy

A clear statement of the scope of the policy is required. This includes a statement outlining the group of people the policy relates to and the group of professionals to whom the policy pertains. In larger or more complex organisations, the policy may refer to specific clinical areas, such as working age adult services in mental health and substance use.

Specific objectives

Stating the specific objectives, and crucial themes, sets out the philosophy that underpins the policy. Objectives may include:

➤ ensuring that individual are not discriminated against due to their lifestyle choices or their needs being perceived as substance induced
➤ delivering care based on need, not diagnosis
➤ providing care from within mainstream services
➤ providing intervention from a multi-agency plan of care with appropriate arrangements for coordinating care
➤ working in a specified service model, e.g. collaborative approach
➤ training and supporting professionals in developing capability.

Definitions

Terms used in the policy need to be defined to provide clarity to all those implementing it. The definition of the individual experiencing mental health–substance use needs agreed locally within the strategy should be included. Other terms such as 'substance use', 'integrated' and 'collaborative working' may require clarification.

Responsibility

A statement regarding responsibility for implementing and adhering to the policy is required to ensure that professionals in the organisation are aware of their duties and accountability.

Processes and procedures

Within the policy, descriptions of processes and procedures are required to specify detailed instructions for professionals in policy implementation.

Staff duties and responsibilities

Referral processes

In keeping with the policy of mainstreaming, people experiencing mental health–substance use needs should access services by the same route as other service users.

Screening and assessment requirements

Setting out arrangements for assessing needs is required to ensure that people receive at least the minimum standard. Specific instructions regarding screening and assessment tools are useful to ensure consistency.

Arrangements for integrated or collaborative working

In this part of the policy, it is useful to show care pathways to illustrate how services and professionals are expected to work together. Arrangements for information sharing can be stated here; usually referring to information-sharing policies within involved organisations as usual processes in mainstream services should apply when working with the individual experiencing mental health–substance use needs.

Systems for planning and coordinating care

It is useful to specify arrangements for agreeing which service is best placed to coordinate care. In areas where care coordination has been the subject of differences of opinion, it may be helpful to state why substance use service are not suitable to lead on the care of individuals requiring secondary mental health services. Moreover, to provide contacts for advice and support on deciding which service is best placed to provide coordination of care.

Clinical structures and specific professional roles

A robust policy requires clear arrangements regarding professional and service structures. The *Dual Diagnosis Good Practice Guide,*[3] suggests a number of possible options for service structures and professionals roles, such as nominating professionals to work between teams and provide clinical leadership. The main duties and roles suggested include:
➤ liaison
➤ training provision
➤ advice
➤ clinical supervision
➤ support.

This embeds the strategy and policy into practice. Findings of the needs assessment will lead commissioners to develop local service plans to address funding and professional arrangements. This frequently involves a combination of funding for specialist, and redesigning existing roles within organisations, such as nominated 'champions' or 'leads'.

Arrangements for training and supporting professionals

The *Dual Diagnosis Good Practice Guide,*[3] advocates development of a training strategy encompassing three strands, or facets, to address the development needs of professionals routinely working alongside individuals experiencing mental health–substance use needs (*see* Box 9.4).

BOX 9.4 The three strands of a training strategy

1 Inter-agency training to develop closer alliances between services.
2 Theoretical and skills-based training.
3 Practice development and supervision to support professionals and embed theoretical training into practice.

Assessing local training requirements during the needs analysis is critical. This basis develops an effective strategy emphasising education, training, and development opportunities tailored to professional needs. Appraising professional mental health–substance use capabilities needs to be formalised through all relevant education, training and appraisal policies and procedures within the organisation to ensure that professionals are reached and their training and development needs addressed. The Dual Diagnosis Capability Framework,[5] provides a useful basis for this.

A coherent policy must set out education and training tailored to the needs of the professional, based upon their role and clinical area. For example, professionals working in Crisis Resolution Services will require education and training in screening and assessment, whereas those working in Assertive Outreach Teams will need to develop skills in delivering interventions, such as motivation and relapse management. Developing a tiered approach to appraising capability education and training ensures that professionals have the level of expertise required. In areas with lower prevalence of mental health–substance use needs, professionals may require awareness-level education and training to develop core capabilities. Professionals who perform a specialised role will require enhanced-level education and training in order to achieve specialist-level capabilities. It is important that professional development does not rely totally on formal education and training. Capabilities can be achieved using a variety of development opportunities, provided through the clinical structure.

Offering appropriate education, training, and development opportunities poses some interesting questions. Is it better to offer academic courses or capability-based development? Can both options be made available? Academic courses can be daunting, and having to be assessed to gain accreditation can deter the professional from attending or completing the course. Professionals who have previously passed academic courses may view further accredited training as unnecessary. Alternatively, for some seeking academic qualifications they may feel that capability-based education and training does not achieve their academic goals.

An arbitration process for resolving differences of opinion

Outlining a system for resolving differences of opinion is an important part of an effective policy and a requirement under the Clinical Negligence Scheme for Trusts.[9] This is due to the need to assist professionals in policy implementation through providing advice and support. A common debate requiring arbitration includes agreeing which service is best placed to provide the role of care co-ordinator or lead professional. Many professionals seek advice and support prior to using the arbitration process in order to check that they have full command of the facts before entering a debate, illustrating why a well-informed lead is a vital part of the support structure. There is also reluctance to use formal processes, such as reporting incidents; many professionals prefer to raise issues informally in order to foster good relationships with other services.

ARRANGEMENTS FOR RESPONDING TO CRISES AND UNTOWARD INCIDENTS

Agreeing arrangements for assessment in crisis can be a lengthy and complex process, as individuals may present to crisis services while under the influence of substances. This can heighten risk and make mental health assessment problematic.

In addition, this heightens anxieties for professionals about their own safety and ability to respond in such situations, generating considerable debate about the role of crisis services in such circumstances. It is important that the consultation process involves hearing the professionals concerns and that policy and procedure addresses these issues. This part of the policy will usually state the need to see the individual to assess risk and determine if a mental health assessment can take place as a minimum standard.

Monitoring and audit arrangements

It is important that there is a statement of how implementation of the policy is monitored within the organisation to ensure that data is collected and reviewed routinely, such as through clinical governance structures. Electronic records may improve ease of access to this information if a single, well-used system is in place. Routine data requirements may have been highlighted during the needs assessment stage of strategy development, particularly information that was not easily accessible at that time. Routine data required may include:

➤ the activity of the professional
➤ referral rates
➤ prevalence, including severity of presenting need
➤ incidents and complaints pertaining to individuals experiencing mental health–substance use needs
➤ education and training activity, evaluation and achievement of capabilities
➤ implementation of the clinical structure.

Specific audit projects may also be useful to examine particular issues.

BOX 9.5 Key steps in policy development

- Senior management in the organisation nominate a lead (or leads) and inform them of the scope of the policy and any relevant deadlines.
- Lead(s) identify representation required to form a working group based upon the clinical and geographical areas to be covered by the policy.
- Leads convene a working group that meets in order to share the remit for the group, agree terms of reference, key tasks, timescale and aims/objectives.
- The group agrees a first draft of the policy and distributes it to selected managers and professionals for a brief targeted consultation to determine whether there are any contentious issues or omissions to resolve before full consultation.
- Comments from the consultation are considered by the group and appropriate changes made prior to the policy being distributed for a formal consultation process.
- The working group is convened to finalise the policy that is then ratified by the organisation and distributed for implementation.

Implementation

Implementing strategy and policy requires consistent leadership and management, with ongoing planning and monitoring through governance structures (*see* Box 9.5). This ensures that strategy and policy documents are not shelved and that their use becomes part of everyday practice. It is important for stakeholders and senior managers to agree an implementation plan with clear objectives and timed targets that impact positively on enhancing the care offered and received by individuals. If the strategy involves a number of stakeholder organisations, the implementation plan will require careful attention regarding who will lead the implementation process in each organisation, and how implementation will be monitored.

Devising meaningful outcome measures is also an important part of the implementation process. Such measures need to reflect the impact on the service user. Useful outcome measures may include:

➤ evidence of implementation of care pathways
➤ screening and assessment of mental health–substance use needs, evidenced in clinical records
➤ integrated care plans incorporating mental health–substance use needs
➤ absence of barriers in accessing services
➤ satisfaction from individuals accessing services
➤ reduction of complaints and incident reports regarding mental health–substance use issues.

LEADING AND MOTIVATING CHANGE AMONG PROFESSIONALS

One of the challenges in developing and implementing strategy and policy is motivation. Compliance with guidance and strategy can be perceived as voluntary and optional. Policies are required to ensure adherence to guidance, as job descriptions and contracts of employment stipulate that organisational policies must be adhered to.

The role of senior management in each organisation is pivotal to the change process. It is essential that they deliver the consistent messages that caring for those with mental health–substance use needs is core business, and that individuals experiencing mental health–substance use problems are already within services, in order to minimise resistance to change.[12]

Promoting an inclusive, whole systems approach that is backed up by formal organisational policy reduces the likelihood of professionals opting out of working with individuals experiencing mental health–substance use problems. However, this does not adequately address negative attitudes to working with these individuals and may be perceived as 'papering over the cracks' in terms of cultural change. While policy provides a formal framework, the need to change 'hearts and minds' remains high priority.

Some professionals may demonstrate resistance to change. This may be due to perceiving the individual experiencing mental health–substance use needs as 'less deserving' or anxieties regarding the professionals own capability.[13] Effective leadership requires insight into the reasons for resistance to change, and how resistance can present. Skills in constructive change management are vital in addressing resistance. The key to effective change management is investing time and support in professionals receptive to change ('early adopters'),[14] who are in positions to be able to influence their peers.

The need for strong, credible leadership when developing and implementing strategy and policy must not be under estimated. A lead is required who has the relevant knowledge, motivation and capability to create meaningful change across diverse services.

CONCLUSION

True mainstreaming of care of people experiencing mental health–substance use needs is not a 'quick fix'. Developing a model that addresses the whole care system including statutory, third sector, and private sector providers requires commitment from professionals, and effective leadership and change management from all levels of the stakeholder organisations. Any policy or strategy documents require drive and ongoing support from senior management and commissioners in order to succeed. Their support and influence is critical to face the challenges and opportunities along the way.

KEY POINTS 9.1

- A whole systems, multi-agency approach will minimise gaps in services.
- As this approach involves a number of organisations, steer and direction from commissioners of services will be required to drive this process.
- The process of engaging and involving stakeholders can be lengthy and complex. However, the time and effort taken is well spent.
- Organisations providing mainstream mental health services require policies and procedures to ensure that professionals provide consistent standards of care.
- Robust implementation plans are required to ensure that strategy and policy is not shelved and ignored. Such plans need to include ongoing monitoring through governance structures.
- Senior managers in stakeholder organisation must be committed to drive implementation.
- The need for consistent, credible leadership is vital.
- Investment in capable lead professional guide the development and implementation of strategies and policies will generate substantial change.

REFERENCES

1 Weaver T, Vikki C, Madden P, *et al*. *Co-morbidity of Substance Misuse and Mental Illness Collaborative Study (COSMIC). Research summaries for providers and commissioners. A study of the prevalence and management of co-morbidity amongst adult substance misuse and mental health treatment populations.* London: National Treatment Agency and Department of Health; 2004. Available at: www.nta.nhs.uk/publications/documents/nta_cosmic_survey_2002_rs1.pdf (accessed 8 June 2010).

2 Department of Health. *National Service Framework*. London: Department of Health; 1999.

3 Department of Health. *Mental Health Policy Implementation Guide: dual diagnosis good practice guide*. London: Department of Health; 2002.

4 Department of Health. *Autumn Assessment Themed Review Report 2007*. London: Department of Health; 2008.

5 Hughes L. *Closing the Gap: a capability framework for working effectively with people with combined mental health and substance use problems (Dual Diagnosis)*. Lincoln: Centre for Clinical and Academic Workforce Innovation, University of Lincoln; 2006.

6 Department of Health. *Dual Diagnosis in Mental Health Inpatient and Day Hospital Settings*. London: Department of Health; 2006.

7 Turning Point. *Dual Diagnosis Good Practice Handbook*. London: Turning Point; 2007.

8 Department of Health. *National Service Framework: five years on*. London: Department of Health; 2004.

9 National Health Service Litigation Authority. *NHSLA Risk Management Standards for Mental Health and Learning Disability Trusts*. National Health Service Litigation Authority; 2009/10. Available at: www.nhsla.com/RiskManagement/ (accessed 8 June 2010).

10 Department of Health. *Refocusing the Care Programme Approach*. London: Department of Health; 2008.

11 Hughes L, Gorry A, Dodd T. *Developing a Capable Dual Diagnosis Strategy*. London: National Mental Health Development Unit; 2009. Available at: www.nmhdu.org.uk/silo/files/developing-a--capable-dual--diagnosis-strategy.pdf (accessed 8 June 2010).

12 Mullins LJ. *Management and Organisational Behaviour*. 6th ed. Harlow: Pearson International-Prentice Hall; 2002.

13 Kotter JP, Cohen DS. *The Heart of Change*. Boston, MA: Harvard Business School Press; 2002.

14 National Health Service Institute for Innovation and Improvement. *Improvement Leaders Guide: managing the human dimensions of change – personal and organisational development*. London: National Health Service Institute for Innovation and Improvement; 2005. Available at: www.institute.nhs.uk/building_capability/building_improvement_capability/improvement_leaders'_guides:_pers.html (accessed 8 June 2010).

TO LEARN MORE

- Centre for Clinical and Academic Workforce Innovation – Tel: +44 (0) 1623 819140 – Email: ccawi@lincoln.ac.uk
- Department of Health – www.dh.gov.uk
- National Health Service Litigation Authority – Tel: +44 (0) 20 7430 8808 – www.nhsla.com
- National Health Service Institute for Innovation and Improvement – Tel: +44 (0) 800 555 550 – www.institute.nhs.uk
- National Treatment Agency – www.nta.nhs.uk
- Turning Point – Tel: +44 (0) 20 7481 7600 – www.turning-point.co.uk

CHAPTER 10

The implications of workplace stress on service development

Philip A Cooper

PRE-READING EXERCISE 10.1

Time: 10 minutes

> 'I just find it very difficult, you know, I mean personally. I find it very difficult that someone does this to themselves . . . they get help for it . . . they get sorted out in hospital and then they go back and do exactly the same thing and put themselves through it all again and again . . . and I have great difficulty with that, because they are so distressed with it.'

This is a quote from an inpatient mental health nurse describing the frustration of dealing with people who come onto the ward after using substances and appear to become mentally unwell again.

- Can you think of any situations where you or colleagues have felt frustration when dealing with people with mental health–substance use problems using substances that impact on their mental health?
- How would you deal with this potentially stressful situation or help other professionals?

After reading this chapter, see if there are any other steps you may take to add to your own solutions.

INTRODUCTION

Health professionals are often hesitant to admit to feeling stressed because of fear of being labelled weak, unable to cope or incapable of professional practice.[1] Substance use among individuals experiencing mental health problems is substantially higher than the general population, with rates as high as 44%–50% in adult inpatient areas.[2,3] Studies have suggested that mental health professionals – in community and inpatient settings – experience high levels of stress and burnout.[4-7] It is a common belief that substance use work is distressing and that professionals are vulnerable to increased psychological morbidity (feelings of tension and alienation from those who use the services) and burnout.[8] The combination of managing both substance use and mental illness can increase the risk of stress and burnout in professionals when addressing these complex challenges.

People with mental health–substance use problems present a number of challenges to professionals trying to address complex needs, and the feelings of families and carers. Individuals experiencing mental health–substance use problems have reported significantly lower family satisfaction, and a greater desire for family treatment.[9] Professionals in hospital settings find that they are in a position where they are likely to experience stressful situations on a daily basis due to individuals using substances. The reason is that substance use is a source of major concern for professionals. The source of this concern includes the use of non-prescribed drugs and alcohol that can increase mental health symptoms and trigger acute illness relapse. Occasionally, it can lead to self-harm or violence to others. Substance use has been viewed as the most common trigger for violence in admission wards.[10] Given the developing nature of the speciality of mental health–substance use problems, together with the associated challenging behaviour, it would seem that working alongside people with mental health–substance use needs will be inherently stressful. This will potentially have a negative impact on developing services and could lead to the provision of ineffective interventions if these stressors are not adequately addressed by the professional, and managers.

In the UK, government legislation requires professionals to maintain a substance-free environment in hospital. However, individuals admitted to hospital may not be ready to stop their substance use. Mental health workers may feel ill-prepared to assess and treat substance use.[11] This can result in a lack of self-esteem, role adequacy and personal achievement leading to increased workplace stress. Professionals can feel uncertain or confused about the effects of substance use, and its interaction with mental ill health.[12] These factors can lead to a lack of effective assessment of substance use.[13] This in turn leads to ineffective interventions. The professionals offering care in these environments can feel frustrated, and experience increased stress levels if individuals continue to use substances and fail to respond to ineffective interventions.[14]

STRESS AND BURNOUT IN THE WORKPLACE

The UK Health and Safety Executive Guide for employees suggest that work-related stress is the adverse reaction a person has to excessive pressure or other types of demand placed upon them.[15] The stressed professional may make mistakes, and put lives at risk. Professionals with unresolved stress may inevitably experience burnout. Professionals with differing individual characteristics may have an increased or decreased chance of developing stress. It appears that reduced levels of self-esteem and personal achievement can lead professionals to increased workplace stress. Burnout is defined as encompassing three elements and can have major impacts on the nature of any treatment or care planning for people experiencing mental health–substance use problems.[16]

1 *The experience of emotional exhaustion* – draining of emotional resources.

2 *Depersonalisation* – developing negative, callous and cynical attitudes towards individuals needing care.
3 *Reduced personal accomplishment* – where there is the tendency to appraise work-related behaviour and performance in a negative manner.

JOB RISK FACTORS IN MENTAL HEALTH AND SUBSTANCE USE SERVICES

Components of work related stress include:
1 factors intrinsic to the job
2 role in the organisation
3 relationships within the work arena
4 career development
5 organisational structure
6 non-work factors.

1 *Factors intrinsic to the job* include stressors, such as having to maintain a substance free environment in hospital or work with individuals who may have a history of violence in the community. Harm minimisation is cited as the most effective intervention for UK substance use services.[17] Paradoxically, mental health professionals in hospital do not have the opportunity to practise harm minimisation. They have to insist on abstinence at the point of admission. However, attempts to force resolution (by enforcing abstinence) can lead to strengthening of the substance use behaviour the professional intends to reduce.
2 *The role of professionals in the organisation* can be confusing as they may wonder whether it is their role to assess and treat substance use. Professionals may feel that substance use work was not what they were trained to do. They were trained to manage mental illness and its treatment, not substance use. The reverse may be true in substance use services.
3 *Relationships with individuals* may be difficult as people who experience mental health–substance use problems have been described as the 'ultimate social monster' in a training resource DVD.[18] Professionals may not be keen to work with potentially unpopular individuals. Professionals may blame the individual for his/her mental health problems because of substances use.
4 *Career development* options may be limited due to the lack of training or preparation to work with mental health–substance use problems. Professionals may be asked to continue their usual role with an interest in substance use (or mental health) problems. Developments in the UK have focused on treating mental health–substance use problems in mainstream mental health services and not as a separate speciality. There is no extra financial incentive to work in a specialist role, working with substance use problems rather than severe mental illness alone. Specific professionals may be perceived as being paid more. This may reduce the incentive and limit career development due to the extra stress of working with complex needs. Working with complex needs without added financial reward, or a defined career development plan in this speciality, may not inspire professionals to work with mental health–substance use problems.

5 *Organisational structure* is important. There has been a lack of strategies to address mental health–substance use problems in health services across the UK.[19] This suggests that in some areas, managers are not supportive and unwilling or unable, to provide resources to help to manage substance use in mental health services effectively.

6 *Non-work factors* include the professional's age in substance use services. Those aged 25 and under have been found to be likely to experience high emotional exhaustion. Substance use professionals experiencing tension, and alienation from individuals, experience increased rates of emotional exhaustion and depersonalisation. Having a supportive partner and greater experience are positive non-work factors that can mediate the effects of work-related stress in the mental health settings.

BURNOUT

Burnout has been associated with a number of stressors. There have been positive correlations between emotional exhaustion and various aspects of care, such as:
➤ violent incidents
➤ continuous one-to-one observations
➤ inadequate staffing
➤ perceived excessive administrative duties and workload.[20]

KEY POINT 10.1

Community professionals find a lack of community facilities to refer on to, work with individuals with a history of violence, and office interruptions major stressors.[21,22]

Professionals identified violence, potential suicide and observation as the most frequent stressors in relation to hospital care.[23] A further study found that ward-based nurses had lost their ability to empathise when compared to community professionals.[24] This loss of empathy could be the result of burnout. It could be concluded that those experiencing the most stress were more likely to:
➤ have increased sick leave
➤ lower self-esteem
➤ feel unfulfilled in their work.[1]

The main stressors for ward-based professionals are inadequate staffing cover in potentially dangerous situations and dealing with health service changes. Professionals in substance use services have cited a number of stressors. These include:
➤ working with demanding individuals
➤ heavy burden of administrative duties
➤ differing organisational demands
➤ shortage of resources
➤ high caseloads
➤ dealing with potentially violent substance using individuals.[25]

These studies relate to professionals in mental health settings dealing with individuals experiencing mental health problems and not specifically mental health–substance use problems. Similarly, the studies in substance use relate to the stressors of working within substance use services. When mental health–substance use problems are prevalent, the stressors for both sets of professionals may be increased in either setting.

WORK-RELATED STRESS AND JOB RISK FACTORS

People experiencing mental health–substance use problems can bring other issues for the professional. It has been suggested that professionals may feel that people experiencing mental health–substance use problems are not popular and engage poorly with services.[26] It could be suggested that some professionals can be angered at being asked to tolerate disturbed behaviour that appears self-induced. In the UK, guidance regarding people experiencing mental health–substance use problems suggested that those who are admitted to hospital can encounter professionals who create sanctions against individuals because they may be seen as being responsible for their own ill health.[27] This could be due to the increased stressors in this environment that result in burnout and depersonalisation. Depersonalisation can result in the development of negative, callous and cynical attitudes towards the individual. This can lead to inappropriate treatment to address substance use as professionals fail to ask about substance use or provide available treatment options.[28] The consequences of these job risk factors are:

➤ higher levels of sick leave
➤ lower self-esteem
➤ Feeling unfulfilled in work
➤ Reduced productivity
➤ Poor morale
➤ Inability to cope.

There are a number of issues that have been highlighted that can contribute to other job risk factors in different services and are summarised in Table 10.1.

TABLE 10.1 Work-related stress job risk factors

	Mental health ward	Mental health community	Substance use services
Violence	✓	✓	✓
Potential suicide	✓		
Administrative duties	✓		✓
Demanding clients			✓
Inadequate staffing/resources	✓		✓
One-to-one observation	✓		
Lack of community facilities		✓	
Organisational changes/demands		✓	✓
Interruptions in the office		✓	
Workload		✓	

MANAGING STRESS FROM MENTAL HEALTH–SUBSTANCE USE PROBLEMS WHEN DEVELOPING SERVICES

When developing services managers need to examine the factors that influence stress levels relating to mental health–substance use. If this is ignored then individuals will not receive effective interventions and treatment. Professionals will view this failure negatively, and empathy will reduce. This may lead to unresolved increasing stressors. The cycle of work-related stress needs to be broken to improve interventions provided to individuals experiencing mental health–substance use problems (*see* Figure 10.1).

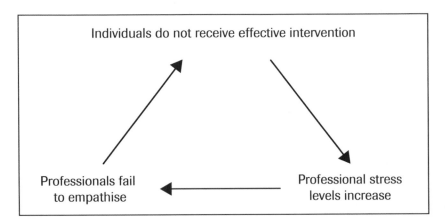

FIGURE 10.1 Cycle of work-related stresses

Six primary areas require specific attention:
1 **Violence and aggression**
   — The issue of aggression and violence is a priority area as substance use is linked with this.[29] Proactive management may enable effective treatment, rather than reacting to incidents as they arise.[30] Early identification and assessment of substance use in mental health settings is vital to begin this process.
   — Asking both professionals and individuals for their views will help the situation and should form the basis of care provision. This enables the development of safer, less stressful working environments.
   — Hospital settings should employ a proactive response to substance use. Before admission to hospital, advance statements or plans from individuals can be extremely useful. This includes actions to be taken if an individual may be tempted to use substances in the abstinent ward environment.
2 **Communication and liaison between services**
   — Encouraging good links with substance use services are a vital component of support for all professionals, who may not feel adequately prepared to deal with mental health–substance use problems.
   — A member of each service attending team meetings in the corresponding service can initially help to break down barriers and build working

alliances. Professionals in services with a specific remit working alongside individuals experiencing mental health–substance use problems require support networks within the organisation, and outside agency support.
— Providing access to professional mentors relating to mental health–substance use enables quality networks that assist in decision-making and teamwork to develop in all services.

3 **Community resources**
— A lack of services when referring on is an issue for all professionals. This requires service developers taking account of the potential lack of community services, and exploring how to meet these community support needs.
— Developing self-help groups or collaborative work with professionals and individuals in the community can improve accessible options.[31] This will allow all involved to discover what support is needed and to provide support in easily accessible/non-stigmatising areas.
— Family interventions in community settings can meet the needs of persons experiencing mental health–substance use problems. This helps to engage the family in accessing support from treatment providers and improves the effectiveness of interventions.

4 **Training initiatives**
— Introducing training initiatives in hospital and the community, and encouraging input from individuals accessing the service to improve interventions, should be vigorously encouraged.

5 **Staffing levels and excessive administrative duties**
— Staffing levels and creative solutions to manage resources and reduce administrative duties need to be urgently addressed when reviewing stressors on professionals.
— Support for the non-qualified professional, who spends more time in intense relationships with individuals due to the extra administrative duties of qualified professionals, must be addressed. Regular support from management should be a priority to improve service provision and reduce stressors.

6 **Clinical supervision**
— Clinical supervision is a formal process of professional support and learning to promote safety of care in complex clinical situations. Providing clinical supervision and mentorship to professionals pro-actively is essential.
— Professionals in mental health teams, including Assertive Outreach Teams or inpatient wards, may find clinical supervision and mentorship essential and indispensable as they deal with a high proportion of individuals experiencing mental health–substance use problems. Effective supervision has been linked to lower levels of burnout in mental health professionals.[32]
— The most important development for improving a service's ability to respond is the appointment of an experienced lead professional. This person, armed with optimism can facilitate natural change in developing services.

CONCLUSION

Mental health–substance use problems present a number of potential stressors to professionals. Recognising these potential stressors, and putting into place strategies that proactively support professionals, and enable individuals to receive the most effective treatment interventions, should be a priority for all those tasked with developing services. The experience of burnout can be alleviated by the availability of coping resources, such as social support.[33] This support can be emotional (clinical supervision/mentorship), or accessing practical support to help solve a work task. The system in the UK fosters service responses that do not routinely address mental health–substance use problems. Managers wishing to develop a needs-led service must acknowledge the issues that prevent effective interventions and treatment. This is maintained by stressors management of all professionals, beginning the process of preventing loss of empathy due to burnout. Reducing work-related stress increases the ability to provide effective interventions.

> We live under threat from painful emotions: anger, desire, pride, jealousy and so on. Therefore we should always be ready to counter these with appropriate antidote. True practitioners may be recognized by their unfailing mindfulness.[34]

SELF-ASSESSMENT EXERCISE 10.1[1] (ANSWERS ON P. 146)

Time: 5 minutes

1 Which of the following are components of 'burnout?'
   a Emotional exhaustion
   b Reduced appetite
   c Loss of libido
   d Depersonalisation
   e Paranoid ideation.

2 Which job factors in healthcare settings contribute to most distress?
   a Poor management
   b Intimacy and death
   c Work overload
   d Role ambiguity
   e Interpersonal problems.

3 Affective signs of work stress include:
   a Tremulousness
   b Early depressions
   c Excessive drinking
   d Chest pain
   e Worry.

4 Accumulated loss phenomena include which of the following:
   a Personal conflict
   b Reduced self-esteem
   c Social withdrawal
   d Agitation
   e Aggression.

REFERENCES

1 Davidson R. Stress issues in palliative care. In: Cooper J, editor. *Stepping into Palliative Care: relationships and responses.* 2nd ed. Oxford: Radcliffe Publishing; 2006.
2 Weaver T, Madden P, Charles V, *et al.* Comorbidity of substance misuse and mental illness

in community mental health and substance misuse services. *Br J Psychiatry.* 2003; **183**: 304–13.

3 Phillips P, Johnson S. Drug and alcohol misuse among inpatients with psychotic illnesses in three inner-London psychiatric units. *Psychiatr Bull.* 2003; **27**: 217–20.

4 Rees D, Smith, S. Work stress in occupational therapists assessed by occupational stress indicator. *Br J Occup Ther.* 1991; **54**: 289–94.

5 Nolan P. A measurement tool for assessing stress among mental health nurses. *Nurs Stand.* 1995; **9**: 36–9.

6 Carson J. Self-esteem and stress in mental health nursing. *Nurs Times.* 1997; **93**: 55–8.

7 McLeod T. Mental health nursing: work stress among community psychiatric nurses. *Br J Nurs.* 1997; **6**: 569–74.

8 Farmer R, Clancy C, Oyefeso A, *et al.* Stress and work with substance misusers: the development and cross-validation of a new instrument to measure staff stress. *Drugs: Educ Prev Polic.* 2002; **9**: 377–88.

9 Dixon L, McNary S, Lehman A. Substance abuse and family relationships of persons with severe mental illness. *Am J Psychiatry.* 1995; **152**: 456–8.

10 Royal College of Psychiatrists, Healthcare Commission. *The National Audit of Violence (2003–2005).* London: HMSO; 2005. p. 1.

11 Renner JA. How to train residents to identify and treat dual diagnosis patients. *Biol Psychiatry.* 2004; **56**: 810–16.

12 Cooper P. Do they know it's drug induced? *Ment Health Nurs.* 2003; **23**: 14–17.

13 Brems C, Johnson ME, Bowers L, *et al.* Comorbidity training needs at a state psychiatric hospital. *Admin Policy Ment Health.* 2003; **30**: 109–20.

14 Deans C, Soar R. Caring for clients with dual diagnosis in rural communities in Australia: the experience of mental health professionals. *J Psychiatr Ment Health Nurs.* 2006; **12**: 268–74.

15 Health and Safety Executive. *Managing the Causes of Work-related Stress: a step-by-step approach using the Management Standards HSG218.* Suffolk: HSE Books; 2007. Available at: www.hse.gov.uk/pubns/books/hsg218.htm (accessed 8 June 2010).

16 Maslach C, Jackson SE. The measurement of experienced burnout. *J Occup Behav.* 1981; **2**: 99–113.

17 Department of Health. *Drug Misuse and Dependence: UK guidelines on clinical management.* London: Department of Health; 2007.

18 Department of Health. *Mental Health Policy Implementation Guidelines: dual diagnosis good practice guide.* London: Department of Health; 2002.

19 Department of Health Care Services Improvement Partnership. *Themed Review Report – Dual Diagnosis.* London: Department of Health; 2008.

20 Jenkins R, Elliot P. Stressors, burnout and social support: nurses in acute mental health settings. *J Adv Nurs.* 2004; **48**: 622–31.

21 Carson J, Bartlett H, Croucher P. Stress in community psychiatric nursing: a preliminary investigation. *Community Psychiatric Nursing Journal.* 1991; **11**: 8–12.

22 Schafer T. CPN Stress and organisational change: a study. *Community Psychiatric Nursing Journal.* 1992; **12**: 16–24.

23 Sullivan PJ. Occupational stress in psychiatric nursing. *J Adv Nurs.* 1993; **18**: 591–601.

24 Fagin L, Brown D, Bartlett H, *et al.* The Claybury community psychiatric nurse stress study; is it more stressful to work in the hospital or the community. *J Adv Nurs.* 1995; **22**: 347–58.

25 Oyefeso A, Clancy C, Farmer R. Prevalence and associated factors in burnout and

psychological morbidity among substance misuse professionals. *BMC Health Services Research.* 2008; **8**: 39, 1–9. Available at: www.ncbi.nlm.nih.gov/pmc/articles/PMC2265695/pdf/1472–6963–8-39.pdf (accessed 8 June 2010).

26 Poole R, Brabbins C. Substance misuse and psychosis. *Br J Hosp Med.* 1997; **58**: 447–50.

27 Department of Health. *Dual Diagnosis in Mental Health Inpatient and Day Hospital Settings.* London: Department of Health; 2006.

28 Barnaby B, Drummond C, McCloud A, *et al.* Substance misuse in psychiatric inpatients: comparison of a screening questionnaire survey with case notes. *Br Med J.* 2003; **327**: 783–4.

29 Phillips P, McKeown O, Sandford T. Dual diagnosis practice in context. Chichester: Wiley-Blackwell; 2010. p. 51.

30 Cooper P, Evans J. Collaborative working – tackling violence, aggression and dual diagnosis. *Ment Health Nurs.* 2007; **27**: 17–20.

31 Cooper P, Fairhurst C, Hill J, *et al.* Drop-in group for dual diagnosis. *Ment Health Nurs.* 2006; **26**: 10–13.

32 Edwards D, Burnard P, Hannigan B, *et al.* Clinical supervision and burnout: the influence of clinical supervision for community mental health nurses. *J Clin Nurs.* 2005; **15**: 1007–15.

33 Melchior MEW, Bours GJJW, Schmitz P, *et al.* Burnout in psychiatric nursing: a meta analysis of related variables. *J Psychiatr Ment Health Nurs.* 1997; **4**: 193–201.

34 Dilgo Khyentse Rinpoche. As cited in: Föllmi D, Föllmi O. *Buddhist Offerings 365 Days.* London: Thames and Hudson.

TO LEARN MORE

- National Consortium of Consultant Nurses in Dual Diagnosis and Substance Use: www.dualdiagnosis.co.uk
- Baker A, Velleman R. *Clinical Handbook of Co-existing Mental Health and Drug and Alcohol Problems.* London: Routledge; 2007.
- Mueser K, Noordsy DL, Drake RE, *et al. Integrated Treatment for Dual Disorders: a guide to effective practice.* New York: Guildford; 2003.
- Edwards D, Burnard P. A systematic review of stress and stress management interventions for mental health nurses. *J Adv Nurs.* 2003; **42**: 169–200.

EXERCISE ANSWERS

ANSWERS TO SELF-ASSESSMENT EXERCISE 10.1

1 a and d
2 b and e
3 b
4 a and b.

CHAPTER 11

Team working

Stephen R Onyett

INTRODUCTION

The UK 2009 New Horizons consultation document on mental health services stated that:

> A key rationale for teams is that they can provide access to the range of specialist skills and expertise necessary to provide a comprehensive assessment of needs and a wide-ranging plan of treatment for people with multiple and complex problems.[1]

People using substance present with a diverse and complex range of health and social care needs that requires the very best that effective team working can deliver.

Figure 11.1, describes team working as a 'holon' or 'whole-part'[2] (combining the Greek 'holos' meaning whole and the suffix 'on' that suggests a particle or part). When thinking of team working it is important to think of it as a whole that represents part of a wider system. It also crucially needs to have as its core the promotion of effective relationships between individuals and professionals. Without that the platform for the assessment and wide range of interventions referred to above and elsewhere in this volume is simply missing. Looking outwards it is crucial that the team connects well with other teams and the wider organisation and promotes connections with the wider range of neighbourhood resources that the individual, as a local citizen, has a right to access. Clearly Figure 11.1 is a gross simplification and this holarchy would need to connect horizontally with other holarchies that form part of ordinary life, such as those concerned with work, education, leisure, the wider local community and society in general.

> **KEY POINT 11.1**
>
> Each level both transcends and includes the levels below and must work to support effective working in that level and the levels it transcends and forms part of.

One author,[3] describes how:

> *work teams include, but are more than (transcend), the sum of interactions between pairs of individuals (dyads); organisational departments include, but are more than, the sum of interactions between teams and dyads; organisations include, but are more than, the sum of interactions between departments, teams and dyads* (p. 271).[3]

It is crucially these interactions, and how we make them more effective, that is the concern in effective team working.

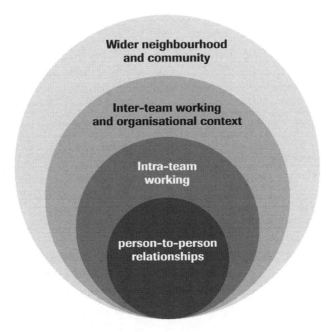

FIGURE 11.1 The teamwork holarchy

WHAT MODEL OF TEAM WORKING FOR MENTAL HEALTH–SUBSTANCE USE?

Box 11.1 describes features of effective team working that pertain to all teams.[4] This chapter will make reference to some of them but focus primarily on those issues that relate most strongly to mental health–substance use.

Of all the different descriptions of teams outlined in the *National Service Framework for Mental Health*,[5] the model that has closest fit with the needs of substance users is assertive outreach. That is not to say that all such teams for serving substance users should become Assertive Outreach Teams or that all the capacity for working effectively with substance users should be located in any kind of specialist team. The more capacity that there is to work effectively with substance use in other parts of the local service system the more flexible and fluid the service

BOX 11.1 The key features of effective team working

- Clear and achievable objectives.
- Differentiated, diverse and clear roles.
- A need for members to work together to achieve shared objectives.
- The necessary authority, autonomy and resources to achieve these objectives.
- A capacity for effective dialogue. This means effective processes for decision-making, being able to engage in constructive conflict and if complex decision-making is involved the team needs to be small enough (no larger than eight or nine people).
- Expectations of excellence.
- Opportunities to review what the team is trying to achieve, how it is going about it and what needs to change.
- Clear and effective leadership.

response is likely to be, and the less likely it is that the individual will be segregated from the mainstream. The *Dual Diagnosis Good Practice Guidelines* (mental health–substance use),[6] advocates:

➤ providing care for mental health–substance use problems within mainstream mental health services through close working with drug and alcohol services

➤ deploying specialist teams of mental health–substance use professionals to provide support to mainstream mental health services

➤ training all professional in Assertive Outreach Teams in work with mental health–substance use, as well as professionals in Crisis Resolution Teams, Early Intervention Teams, inpatient services and Community Mental Health Teams

➤ ensuring that care coordination extends to people experiencing mental health–substance use problems and all the services that work with them.

Assertive Outreach Teams should already include people experiencing mental health–substance use problems within their remit, and are designed to focus on motivation, and the need to match level of engagement with the mode of provision supplied. They have more capacity to work with people who are more likely to have unstable living accommodation and contact with the criminal justice system. In that Assertive Outreach Teams increasingly focus on the younger population, with higher expectations of community integration and self-determination, they may also provide a less segregated service. Moreover, there is evidence that the model is effective.[7,8]

Assertive outreach crucially emphasises the establishment of effective working relationships between individuals and professionals. This is perhaps the only way in which underlying feelings about substance use and the place of substance use in the individual's life may surface. Like most individuals, people using substances want to be listened to, and heard. In time, this can also create opportunities to explore key historical aspects of the individual's development of substance use, for example previous experience of violence or abuse. Longer-term involvement also allows for complex interactions to be observed and learned from, for example in terms of the effects of complex interactions between prescribed and non-prescribed drugs.

Assertive outreach practice: key features

➤ Efforts to achieve effective engagement both with the team and other services.
➤ Being proactive in providing practical support and assistance.
➤ Giving time.
➤ Reflecting the demographic characteristics of the locality, the life experience of the individual, and promoting choice. 'New Horizons',[1] highlights the value of employing professionals who have had personal experiencing with using substances as a way of promoting a service that is more responsive to need.
➤ Providing relevant services. Bristol MIND's (England) 'user-lead study' of Assertive Outreach Teams highlighted that people were not intrinsically 'hard to engage' but rather simply did not see that what was on offer was relevant to them.[9] Often this will include a focus on housing, occupation and money.
➤ An ability to work with or for individuals, rather than making plans on their behalf.
➤ Persistence. Up to six months devoted to developing a therapeutic alliance.
➤ Commitment to long-term relationships, over at least 12 months but often many years.
➤ The right 'style'– perhaps as informed by their life experience.
➤ Low expressed emotion – non-critical, non-judgemental, and accepting, including accepting a certain level of risk.
➤ Ability to work with individuals in informal settings including working in the individuals social environment, where appropriate, and where they and the professional (unqualified and qualified) feel safe to do so. By working as much in context as possible, the individual's wider context is effectively considered in the work.
➤ Flexibility with respect to working hours and activities undertaken.
➤ Knowledge about services in the community, covering both the range and quality of providers.
➤ An understanding of the working of local authorities, benefits and housing agencies, health and social care provision and the voluntary sector.
➤ Working as intensively as required, with the capacity to visit several times a week if necessary.
➤ Not time limited.
➤ Available 24 hours a day, or at the very least have a very strongly coordinated and seamless approach to working with other out-of-hours teams.
➤ Focus on provision rather than just brokering referrals to other agencies.
➤ Responsibility maintained regardless of who else is involved. The team should serve to integrate different inputs rather than just collect more.
➤ Limited caseloads.
➤ Individually focused education, support, treatment and therapy.
➤ Emphasis on monitoring and review.

REFLECTIVE PRACTICE EXERCISE 11.1

> **Time: 10 minutes**
> Reviewing the bullet points above, how does the team that you know best compare.
> First of all run through the list highlighting from 1 to 5 how important that feature
> of team practice is in your opinion, with 1 representing 'Not important at all' to 5
> meaning 'Absolutely crucial'.
>   Now run through again, this time rating where you feel your team is now from
> 1 to 5, where 5 is 'We are brilliant at this' and 1 is 'We don't do this at all.'
> Now subtract the second number from the first (you might get some negative
> numbers, e.g. 2 − 5 = −3). What does this tell you about where to direct some
> attention?

THE TEAM APPROACH

In a pure assertive outreach model there is value placed on a 'team approach',
whereby all individuals are expected to have a relationship with all team professionals, rather than a single professional in a care coordinator or key-worker role.
Some of the advantages claimed for this approach include:

➤ improved continuity of care because strong relationships with professionals
  have not come and gone
➤ reliable weekly contact because workloads are shared
➤ opportunities for more intensive and flexible responses as professionals can be
  called upon to respond to changing need
➤ a better response to crises that is not reliant on one professional's availability;
➤ better peer support and consultation
➤ reduced stress for professionals, partly because of the greater containment of
  the emotional responses
➤ better access for individuals experiencing mental health–substance use
  problems to professionals who may share or be sensitive to their unique
  cultural and ethnic background
➤ the avoidance of 'pathological dependency' whereby the professionals ability
  to improve the mental health of the individual paradoxically reinforces their
  low selfesteem, and sense of inadequacy and personal failure. It has been
  reported that far from always being 'pathological', their experience suggested
  that periods of dependence are part of a normal pathway to independence.[10]

There is some evidence for effective engagement among individuals, and good
morale among professionals in teams, using this approach.[11] However, there are
major downsides. Some individuals have a preference for individual relationships with fewer professional.[11] One study,[12] identified difficulties *'for any human
being to establish warm, supportive, and trusting relationships with a team'* (p. 7).[12]
Similarly, another study,[10] found it problematic in working with people who were
mistrustful.

    Many teams claiming adherence to the team approach in reality operate more
flexibly in response to need.[10] The most pragmatic and sensitive response is usually

to consider the individuals, and their social networks, as the centre of the team and build the required supports and relationships around them on the basis of their preferences, needs and experience of what works. Building up one relationship through time, commitment and consistency, and only then working to expand the network of professionals involved, so that at least three members of the team are fully familiar with the individual.[10]

REFLECTIVE PRACTICE EXERCISE 11.2

> **Time: 5 minutes**
> Based on your knowledge of this individual group where do you feel that your team should be on this continuum from purely individual case working to a full-blown team approach where individual more exclusive relationships are frowned upon? Where are you in practice? Do you need to make any changes?

GENERIC OR SPECIALISED PROFESSIONALS?

The exact opposite of the team approach is the 'generic' key-worker approach where one professional supplies all one-to-one contact. In practice, if the individual really needs contact with only one team professional, then they probably do not need to be seen by a team at all. The more generic approach was characteristic of the 'all things to all people' ideology of some community mental health centres of the late 1980s, where valued notions of democratic team structures and flat hierarchies served to fudge the need to examine individual practice, skill mix within the team, and individual team members' different levels of authority to make decisions. In effect those with the most complex needs lost out.[13]

Effective teams have clear and shared objectives and are staffed by professionals in differentiated, diverse and clear roles where each can see the contribution that they make to the aims of the team as a whole. These differentiated roles are accompanied by a need among members to work together to achieve team objectives.[14] If this interdependency is not there to meet the complex range of needs presenting, then it is questionable whether a team is needed.

KEY POINT 11.2

Although diversity is a key feature of effective teams, some aspects of everyone's roles will be shared among team members. This might include:
- processes for communications – record-keeping
- how core assessments are undertaken
- how risk is managed
- how case reviews are undertaken.

This helps team members maintain a high level of awareness of each other's workload.

WORKING APPRECIATIVELY TOWARDS BETTER DIALOGUE

The phrase 'working appreciatively' is a shorthand for an approach that specifically focuses on appreciating the positive that individuals bring to a situation. Guidelines on assertive outreach stress the need to focus on at least one aspect of the individual that can be viewed positively and focused on, regardless of disturbed or challenging behaviour. This includes:

➤ their personal strengths and resources
➤ the value of what they have done already
➤ particularly actions that (either in themselves, or in the outcomes they produce) are in some way like the preferred future those individuals describe for themselves.

In that this solution-focused approach appears to be effective at a clinical level,[15] it seems fruitful to explore how such principles might play out at different levels within systems (*see* Figure 11.1). The application of solution-focused thinking to organisations[16] and 'appreciative inquiry' are organisational interventions that consciously seek out and express people's best resources, assets and intentions.[17,18]

This is important at both a clinical, intra-team and inter-team level. For professionals to exercise the non-judgement approach that is required for effective working, they need to be able to exercise and receive such non-judgemental and affirming relationships from colleagues, managers and leaders. It has been highlighted[19] how the majority of nurses became involved in this work because of a specific interest in these individuals and their problems. It is argued that greater emphasis should be placed on this attribute when selecting new employees.[19] This also needs to be given expression with professionals finding opportunities to express, through words and deeds, the best values that they bring to the job, and for other professionals to notice, and provide some affirmation. This is not just about being nice. There is considerable evidence that the creation of a 'positive emotional climate' at work is associated with better outcomes on a range of measures.[20]

Part of taking a non-judgemental approach within the team includes working well with different ideologies of care. One study[21] identified a problem with authoritarian attitudes among consultants, and a frustration among other professionals that the 'medical model', in tending to view substance use as harmful and detrimental to mental states, was in conflict with the view of the individual.[22] An approach is needed where the individual is met on their own turf both literally and metaphorically. Being non-judgemental is not about denying your own feelings about substance use. It is around being self-aware of what they are, and how this might be received and perceived by the individual. As in any relationship, being authentic is important for all parties.

Exhortation to be different is ineffective, and professionals need to respectfully consider the pros and cons of change, and no-change for individuals. For example, in stopping substance use, an individual may lose contact with a social network that has benefits for them. The team needs to work with the individual on what is needed to fill that gap, and maximising the creativity of the team is crucial. In many contexts, this means that the emphasis is on harm minimisation rather than cessation and abstinence.

None of this means that the team should adopt a uniform ideology. Indeed, rather than focussing on areas of commonality that precludes new solutions emerging, the communications within the team should instead value diversity, and thus the fuller universe of solutions that might emerge. At best, teams should aim for a deep dialogue (*see* Bohm[23]) to emerge where team members are able to suspend assumptions and judgements, and promote active and attentive listening and personal and collective reflection on the thoughts and ideas that emerge. Conflict is valuable as long as it does not become personalised or persecutory, or the exercise of illegitimate power relationships in play within the team.[24] Creating a bedrock of appreciative working may prevent this. Contrary to popular wisdom, it is not always crucial to resolve 'relationship' conflicts, unless of course one party is subject to oppressive or bullying behaviour. Collaboratively managing new task conflicts while ignoring interpersonal annoyances may sometimes be beneficial in facilitating team working.[25]

KEY POINT 11.3

The desire to do good work is one important shared value that transcends interpersonal differences.

It is important to acknowledge that while a team may be thinking about long-term goals with respect to work with individuals, that person may be living, deciding and choosing minute by minute. Nonetheless, a good working formulation of how the individual's current issue emerged and what precedes and maintains problematic behaviours will be needed.[26] This forms the basis of collaborative work on small next steps to a preferred future.

Although diversity is invaluable, team members must have shared social reality about what they are doing, and a shared language with which to describe this reality. Building this shared reality should start with the experience of the individual, and language that promotes their inclusion. A mature team with stable membership is better placed to develop members who can take the perspective of others into account in relation to both their emotional and cognitive position. In these circumstances, the team is better able to recognise the source of communication difficulties when they arise.

There needs to be a recognisable and agreed process for communication and decision-making. It is important that decision-making is visible, inclusive and coherent, and that it is afforded time and substance (*see* To learn more).

INTER-TEAM WORKING

People experiencing mental health–substance use problems are often stigmatised, with the fact of their substance use serving as a barrier to their being readily accepted by other services.[27,28] When substance use is raised, people often stop listening. One study,[21] found that the reputations of individuals experiencing mental health–substance use problems meant that agencies and organisations were reluctant to provide necessary resources. Housing was a particular problem. Nurses reported that general practitioners' participation in services was inconsistent forcing some nurses to take undue responsibility for clinical decision-making.[19] Some Crisis and Home Treatment Teams, which are supposed to provide the final common pathway to acute inpatient care often, either explicitly or implicitly, exclude people with substance use problems, despite the very high prevalence of substance use in inpatient environments. It was found that individuals experiencing mental health–substance use problems:

➤ needed more crisis intervention
➤ were less likely to take prescribed medication
➤ were unpredictable in attending appointments (hence again the need for an assertive outreach focus)
➤ had more hospital admissions than individuals with mental health problems alone.

For this reason, they require sophisticated and effective responses with respect to how the team connects to other parts of the local service system.

There is a natural and universal tendency to form groups that define themselves partly through denigration of other groups. This forms the bedrock of much of the stereotyping and impaired inter-group working that undermines partnership working at all levels. In tackling this, one study,[29] highlighted the role of boundary spanners, often the team manager, who have a dual identity – a positive sense of belonging to both the team and the wider organisation or service. They found this dual identity was positively related to effective inter-group relations, particularly if they had frequent contact with other groups. Their identification with the bigger picture appeared to function as a buffer against the detrimental effects of group identification by shifting the focus to the larger group without blurring team boundaries. Whilst appreciating the bigger picture, it was important that the team could see how it made its own particular contribution to the aims of the service as a whole. Managers could combat ineffective intergroup relations by enhancing employees' identification with their organisation while acknowledging teams for their individual performance.[29] Measures for enhancing organisational identification include:

➤ communication of organisational successes, values, and goals
➤ rotation of individual boundary spanners into key roles
➤ promotion into boundary positions of employees with dual identification
➤ ensuring inter-group working, frequent inter-group meetings and inter-group social gatherings are on the team's agenda.

REFLECTIVE PRACTICE EXERCISE 11.3

Time: 5 minutes

Think about the team that you have most difficulty working with and that you feel your team needs to work more effectively with in the interests of individuals. How could you go about getting to know that team better?

TEAM LEADERSHIP

Team leadership is about creating a supportive environment for creative thinking, for challenging assumptions about how the service should be delivered. It is also about sensitivity to the needs of a range of internal and external stakeholders, inside and outside the team and the organisation. Managers of front-line professionals must be visible, and available to, professionals, and accountable for service delivery.[30]

Working appreciatively within the team, and across teams, and indeed with individuals is something that needs to be modelled by the team leader. Effective managers of Community Mental Health Teams constantly modelled good practice.[31] They tended to focus less on traditional features of management, such as attending meetings, preparing reports and proposals, and instead spent most of their time helping individuals or professionals to achieve their goals. This chimes strongly with recent research on team management that stresses that the single most important leadership quality for predicting professionals' productivity and service outcomes was the capacity to engage with others and, in particular, to show personal concern for the welfare and aspirations of the person they line managed.[32]

There are some practical contextual issues that only leaders and managers at team level and above can address. For example, when looking at the whole local service context it is important that individual pathways to, through and from team-based provision have clear and dedicated capacity to work with these individuals. There is a need for the local service system to map demand and capacity. This individual group should have the same access to the care programme approach and effective risk management processes as the rest of the population served. Inclusion and exclusion criteria that teams adopt when looked at holistically within a locality should make explicit how people experiencing substance use problems will be served. Otherwise, they are likely to find themselves 'bounced' around the local service, which is devaluing, creates further disaffection, and works against effective engagement with local services. Where people are 'bounced' this should be audited and reported to service commissioners.[33] These problems remains as true for rural as for urban contexts.

There is the issue of who should lead the team. As the *New Ways of Working for Psychiatrists* report states (p. 46) (*see* www.newwaysofworking.org.uk):

> *Clearly no discipline can claim to have exclusive competences for* [team leadership] *as a consequence of their professional training. Individuals from all professional backgrounds need to be developed and selected with care to fulfil these crucial team management/leadership roles* (p. 46).[34]

The wide range of knowledge, skills and experience among disciplines within the team means that an open, transparent and equitable approach is needed to determine leadership roles that are not overly influenced by the social value attached to particular disciplines. Ultimately, the job of the leader is to create an environment wherein everyone can exercise leadership to the full extent of their power and authority, including the individual. However, it is important that formal leadership roles are clear, and that there is an absence of conflict about leadership. This is associated with leadership clarity that in turn is associated with:

> ➤ clear team objectives
> ➤ high levels of participation
> ➤ commitment to excellence
> ➤ support for innovation.[35]

THE NEED FOR PERSONAL SUPPORT

A primary feature of team working is the need for participative safety, in other words the capacity of the team to welcome contributions from all team members (e.g. in meetings) without their being any fear of ridicule or abuse.[35] Professionals are at particular risk of feeling deskilled when working with people experiencing mental health–substance use problems.[21] The work is stressful not only because of the nature of the individuals presentations but also because of organisational issues including:

> ➤ changes in services
> ➤ funding issues
> ➤ lack of education and training
> ➤ lack of support.[36,37]

It is crucial that the team defends time to review its internal processes, including maintaining awareness of all its strengths and assets. Moreover, the ways in which energy and creativity can be maintained through people feeling able to contribute to their best even when ideas may seem tentative or 'half-baked'.

CONCLUSION

Teams are part of wider systems comprising human beings in relationship with each other. It should therefore not surprise us that what works well at a clinical level, also informs what we should be doing as leaders, managers and team members at every other level. As people we need to feel heard and on the end of authentic personal concern from others. Our needs should be properly assessed and responded to in a way that makes full use of our diverse talents and resources, experience of when we are at our best, and our highest aspirations.

REFERENCES

1 Department of Health. *New Horizons: towards a shared vision for mental health*. Consultation. London: Mental Health Division; 2009.

2 Koestler A. *The Ghost in the Machine*. London: Arkana; 1967.

3 Edwards MG. The integral holon: a holonomic approach to organisational change and transformation. *J Org Change Manag*. 2005; **18**: 269–88.

4 Onyett SR. *Working Psychologically in Teams*. Leicester: British Psychological Society/ National Institute of Mental Health in England; 2007.

5 Department of Health. *National Service Framework for Mental Health: modern standards and service models*. London: Department of Health; 1999. Available at: www.dh.gov.uk/ en/Publicationsandstatistics/Publications/PublicationsPolicyAndGuidance/DH_4009598 (accessed 8 June 2010).

6 Department of Health. *Mental Health Policy Implementation Guide: dual diagnosis good practice guide*. London: Department of Health; 2002. Available at: www.substance misuserct.co.uk/staff/documents/dh_4060435.pdf (accessed 8 June 2010).

7 Drake RE, McHugo GJ, Clark RE, *et al*. Assertive community treatment for patients with co-occurring severe mental illness and substance use disorder: a clinical trial. *Am J Orthopsychiatry*. 1998; **68**: 201–15.

8 Department of Health. *Assertive Outreach in Mental Health in England: report from a day seminar on research, policy and practice*. London: Department of Health; 2005. Available at: http://kc.csip.org.uk/upload/AO%20seminar%20report.pdf (accessed 8 June 2010).

9 Davies R, Shocolinsky-Dwyer R, Mowat J, *et al*. *Effective Involvement in Mental Health Services: assertive outreach and the voluntary sector*. Bristol: Bristol Mind; 2009. Available at: www.bristolmind.org.uk (accessed 8 April 2010).

10 Burns T, Firn M. *Assertive Outreach in Mental Health: a manual for practitioners*. Oxford: Oxford University Press; 2002.

11 Gauntlett N, Ford R, Muijen M. *Teamwork: models of outreach in an urban multi-cultural setting*. London: Sainsbury Centre for Mental Health; 1996.

12 Spindel P, Nugent JA. *The Trouble with PACT: questioning the increasing use of assertive community treatment teams in community mental health*. 1999. Available at: www.peoplewho. org/readingroom/spindel.nugent.htm (accessed 8 June 2010).

13 Patmore C, Weaver T. Unnatural selection, *Health Serv J*. 1991; **101**: 20–2.

14 Carter AJ, West MA. Sharing the burden: teamwork in health care settings. In: Payne R, Firth-Cozens J, editors. *Stress in Health Professionals: psychological and organisational causes and interventions*. Chichester: Wiley; 1999. pp. 191–202.

15 de Shazer S, Dolan Y, Korman H, *et al*. *More than Miracles: The state of the art of solution-focused brief therapy*. New York: Haworth Press; 2007.

16 Jackson PZ, McKergow M. *The Solutions Focus*. London: Nicholas Brealey Publishing; 2002.

17 Cooperrider DL, Whitney D, Stavros J. *Appreciative Inquiry Handbook: The first in a series of AI workbooks for leaders of change*. Bedford Heights, OH: Lake Shore Communications; 2003.

18 Hammond SA. *The Thin Book of Appreciative Inquiry*. 2nd ed. Bend, OR: Thin Book Publishing; 1998.

19 Grafham E, Matheson C, Bond CM. Specialist drug misuse nurse's motivation, clinical decision-making and professional communication: an exploratory study. *J Psychiatr Ment Health Nurs*. 2004; **11**: 690–7.

20 Ozcelik H, Langton N, Aldrich H. Doing well and doing good: the relationship between leadership practices that facilitate a positive emotional climate and organizational performance. *J Manag Psycholy*. 2008; **23**: 186–203.

21 Coombes L, Wratten A. The lived experience of community mental health nurses working with people who have dual diagnosis: a phenomenological study. *J Psychiatr Ment Health Nurs*. 2007; **14**: 382–92.

22 Phillips P. The mad, the bad and the dangerous – harm reduction in dual diagnosis. *Int J Drug Policy*. 1998; **9**: 345–9.

23 Bohm D. On dialogue. In: Nichol L, editor. *The Essential David Bohm*. London: Routledge; 1996.

24 Pelled LH. Demographic diversity, conflict, and work group outcomes: an intervening process theory. *Organ Sci*. 1995; **7**: 615–31.

25 De Dreu CK, Van Vianen AE. Managing relationship conflict and the effectiveness of organisational teams. *J Organ Behav*. 2001; **22**: 309–28.

26 Johnstone L, Dallos R, editors. *Formulation in Psychology and Psychotherapy: making sense of people's problems*. London: Routledge; 2006.

27 Rassool GH. Addiction: global problem and global response. Complacency or commitment? *J Adv Nurs.* 2000; **32**: 505–7.

28 Hipwell A, Singh K, Clark A. Substance misuse among individuals with severe and enduring mental illness: service utilisation and implications for clinical management. *J Ment Health.* 2000; **9**: 37–50.

29 Richter AW, West MA, Van Dick R, *et al.* Boundary spanners' identification, intergroup contact, and effective intergroup relations. *Acad Manage J.* 2006; **49**: 1252–69.

30 Sainsbury Centre for Mental Health. *Keys to Engagement.* London: Sainsbury Centre for Mental Health; 1998.

31 Gowdy E, Rapp CA. Managerial behaviour: the common denominator of effective community-based programs. *Psychosoc Rehabil J.* 1989; **13**: 31–51.

32 Alimo-Metcalfe B, Alban-Metcalfe J, Bradley M, *et al.* The impact of engaging leadership on performance, attitudes to work, and well-being at work: A longitudinal study. *J Health Organ Manag.* 2008; **22**: 586–98.

33 Clark J. *'On the Bounce'. Understanding Mental Health Systems in the North West.* Care Services Improvement Partnership; 2008. Available at: www.northwest.nhs.uk/document _uploads/Mental_Health_in_the_North_West/On_the_Bounce_Report.pdf (accessed 8 June 2010).

34 Department of Health. *New Ways of Working for Psychiatrists: enhancing effective, person-centered services through new ways of working in multidisciplinary and multia-gency contexts.* London: Department of Health; 2005. Available at: www.dh.gov.uk/en/ Publicationsandstatistics/Publications/PublicationsPolicyAndGuidance/DH_4122342 (accessed 8 June 2010).

35 West MA, Markiewicz L. *Building Team-based Working: a practical guide to organizational transformation.* Oxford: Blackwell Publishing; 2004.

36 McMillan I. Ordinary people, extraordinary problems. *Nurs Stand.* 1997; **11**: 19–20.

37 Farmer R, Clancy C, Oyefeso A. Stress amongst substance misuse professionals. *Substance Misuse Bulletin.* 1999; **12**: 9.

TO LEARN MORE

This chapter has only scratched the surface of a wide ranging subject. For a comprehensive review of some of the primary issues with respect to team working *see*:

- The *Working Psychologically in Teams* document at: www.bps.org.uk document-download-area/document-download$.cfm?file_uuid=12B7C9B9-1143-DFD0-7E1C-75AEDF90F941 &ext=pdf

For detail of teamwork issues, including team design, process and leadership *see*:

- Onyett SR. *Teamworking in Mental Health.* London: Palgrave; 2003.

For a scholarly review of a range of teamwork issues *see*:

- Byrne M. A response to the Mental Health Commission's discussion paper 'Multidisciplinary Team Working: from theory to practice'. *The Irish Psychologist.* 2006; **32**: 323–39. See also the same author's guidance on team working written for the Irish Mental Health Commission.

For recent guidance on responsibility and accountability issues *see*:

- The National Institute for Mental Health in England National Workforce Programme. *Moving*

On: From new ways of working to a creative capable workforce – guidance on responsibility and accountability. 2009. Available at: www.newwaysofworking.org.uk/

For issues concerning team training *see*:

- The Creating Capable Teams Approach. Available at: www.newwaysofworking.org.uk

For the effective Teamworking and Leadership Programme *see*:

- Onyett SR, Rees A, Borrill C, *et al.* The evaluation of a local whole systems intervention for improved team working and leadership in mental health services. *The Innovation Journal.* 2009. Available at: www.innovation.cc/scholarly-style/onyett6.pdf

For tools for evaluating the effectiveness of your team working *see*:

- The Integrated Team Monitoring and Assessment. However, I would not advocate using such tools outside of an affirming solution-focused development process, otherwise people may merely assess their team as poor and become demoralised: www.readiness-tools.com/tool-full.aspx?toolguid=0d6382ad-f017–4623–8d10–93f2f314e346
- The Aston Team Performance Inventory. Available at: www.astonod.com/atpiView.php?page=1
- The Community Mental Health Team Effectiveness Questionnaire. See Rees A, Stride C, Shapiro DA, *et al.* Psychometric properties of the Community Mental Health Team effectiveness questionnaire. *J Ment Health.* 2001; **10**: 213–22.
- The Productivity Measurement and Enhancement System: http://promes.cos.ucf.edu/index.php

For more on working appreciatively and with a solution focus *see*:

- The Centre for Solution Focus at Work. Available at: www.sfwork.com
- A very rich source of Solution Focus papers and presentations from around the world: www.solworld.org
- Home of the work of Cooperrider, the founder of the Appreciative Inquiry approach: http://appreciativeinquiry.case.edu/
- Good source of publication details at Appreciative Inquiry at University of Virginia: http://appreciativeinquiry.virginia.edu

CHAPTER 12

Communication: the essence of good practice, management and leadership

David B Cooper

. . . about courtesy and good manners . . .

> **Time: 30 minutes**
> Consider the following:
> 1 When was the last time you wished communication within or outwith your team could be improved?
> 2 What steps do you think you could take to improve the communication?

INTRODUCTION

'*Effective . . . communication is a master key . . . it fits all locks and opens all doors to therapeutic treatment and intervention.*'[1] However, if communication is pivotal: why do we often get it wrong? If effective communication is easy: why do we not practice it all the time? If we are pleased when communication has gone well and angry when it has not: why do we have high expectations of other's effective communication and not pay attention to our own?

As individuals, we should know *what to do* and *how to do it* – there are no excuses. Yet, we remain ineffective communicators – unless it impacts on us directly. Then we become experts – we notice how *ineffective* communication damages our day!

Here we provide a foundation for common courtesy and good practice that should be part of our professional and personal lives. We have become too familiar with poor communication and easily over-simplify or underestimate its importance. Consequently, we miss the value it holds for individuals, groups and ourselves.

Table 12.1 offers the definition for key words used in this chapter.

TABLE 12.1 Definitions

Word	Definition
Communicate	To impart (knowledge) or exchange (thoughts) by speech, writing, gesture, etc.[2]
	To share information with others by speaking, writing, moving your body, using signals[3]
Communication	The imparting or exchange of information, ideas or feelings[2]
Effective	Productive of or capable of producing a result[2]
Intra-	Within, inside[2]
Inter-	Between, mutually, together, reciprocally[2]

WHAT IS EFFECTIVE COMMUNICATION?

Communication can be subdivided into seven parts.
1 *Individual, family and carers.*
2 *Junior team.*
3 *Peers.*
4 *Intra-disciplinary team.*
5 *Inter-disciplinary team.*
6 *Middle management.*
7 *Senior management.*

Each is interdependent and interrelated – none stands alone.

Integral to, and at the centre of all the professionals' actions, is effective communication with the individual, family and carers. It is they who experience the negative consequence of ineffective communication. Therefore, effective communication is like the ripples in a pond, flowing effortlessly between each part.

What is the communication pond?

Water is made up of millions of individual molecules which collectively give water its fluidity. Individuals within an organisation, or interlinked fields, are like the individual molecules of water. Each is interdependent on the other to provide the best possible quality standard of care for the individual, family and carers.

Imagine a stone landing in a pond. The ripples move seamlessly through the water until the pond is smooth, ready for the next stone. In this analogy, *you* are the stone – represented by *ME* in Figure 12.1. The *ME* is placed anywhere in the organisational structure. Wherever *you* are in the chart *ME* is the centre for effective communication. It is *your* responsibility to ensure *your* communication flows effectively and effortlessly through the organisation.

Therefore, effective communication emanates like the ripples on a pond, flowing effortlessly. Each professional having an equal responsibility to effectively communicate with the other: each intra- and inter-dependent. Only then can communication – and the care of the individual, family and carers – be effective.

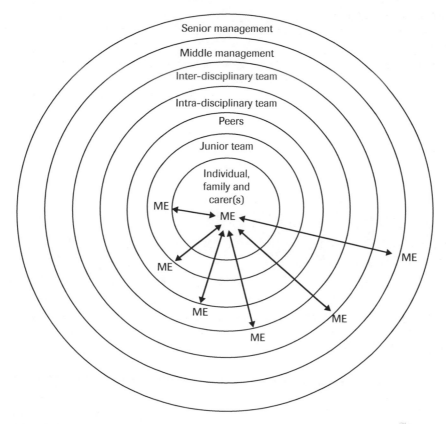

FIGURE 12.1 Communication pond

1 Individual, family and carers

The individual, family and carers are central in any care environment. Every action, act or omission, from the junior member to the most senior manager, impacts on these individuals. Ineffective communication makes the treatment and intervention experience devastating and destructive.

The impact of verbal communication between professionals cannot be overemphasised. How professionals share important and routine information related to the individual, family and carers, does have a major impact on the successful outcome of any therapeutic intervention.

With the individual's permission, information relating to past and present health or social problems can be discussed with each professional or agency. Just as important, is the information available from family/carers relating to the individual's concerns. The individual may forget or be unable to express important facts and information relevant to the presenting problem. Often, individuals and family can feel intimidated by the knowledgeable professional.

The individual, family and carers can become dependent on the professional. This is not a deliberate act. It is easy to feel *safe* in the hands of a competent professional. The individual comes to depend on *immediate* access and, consequently, sudden unexpected and unplanned withdrawal is disruptive. The individual, family and carers should be informed at the outset about the level and extent of your involvement in their care. This should be periodically reinforced so the individual is aware of *your* end-date.

Moreover, it is possible for the professional to extend contact with the individual, family and carers beyond that which is therapeutic. We gain subconscious reward from their dependence on us – the professional! Clinical supervision aids identification of over-involvement and dependence. Individuals do progress without our watchful eye if appropriate and effective intervention and treatment is managed effectively. We cannot protect them from all ills or dangers. Being aware of one's limitations, intervention and the extent of the therapeutic value, takes experience. Close monitoring of our actions is essential. A good marker is when we come to write the legal records related to the individual and we have little to say about the person's progress – it is time to evaluate ones effectiveness. Ineffective communication is damaging and destructive.

2 Junior team

Students and junior team members often feel isolated from the communication loop. Matters involving the organisation are heard on the grapevine, often half-factual, sometime totally inaccurate. Effective communication with junior members of the team is just as important as in any other area of the organisation. Unease and job dissatisfaction arise when the individual feels that he/she is unheard.

New employees are often unsure of the system and reluctant to express ideas and concepts for fear of reprimand or being labelled as trouble-makers. Old hands do not always have the best or brightest concepts. Communication *among and between* junior team members and senior colleagues should be actively encouraged. Where possible, new ideas and initiatives should be given a fair hearing and encouraged. Yes, it may be that '*it has been tried before and failed*' but maybe the time was not right or indeed the motivation. With supervision, support and encouragement, junior team members bring new ideas to the fore that can improve care and communication.

Why is he/she doing this?

The easiest way to germinate suspicion and misunderstanding is to issue a directive that has no prior or present explanation as to its use. For example, statistics – in any format – are the bane of many. Without careful explanation of the value of new statistic collection (i.e. to ensure that the service is adequately resourced and funded), suspicion can evolve to a negative response. '*Don't they think I am working hard enough?*' '*Why are they watching me?*' An explanation offsets the misconception, maintains productivity and improves working practice. Explanations of complex or role-changing information should be *face-to-face*. It is *not* acceptable to email or send a memorandum – this is, at the least, bad manners and poor practice.

3 Peers

Communication upwards: managers are not clairvoyant – tell them!

A common complaint from team members is that the manager does not understand them. Like the manager, we, as individuals have a responsibility to communicate.

Managers do not come to the post with a vacuum-packed crystal ball; nor are they clairvoyant – even if the issues seem blatantly obvious to you. Nor do they know everything there is to know about the workforce as a managerial tribal birthright. The manager needs clear and concise feedback. It is no use complaining that the manager does not appreciate the needs of your job, or that one is working in excess of one's designated hours, if this is not explained to him or her. Likewise, it is no use complaining about the excessive workload and yet still work the excess hours for fear that this might jeopardise treatment, care and interventions: *as professionals, we have a responsibility to communicate effectively too!* Moreover, you support your complaint with statistics!

One cannot place all of the responsibility for ineffective communication on the boss! Each individual is capable of demonstrating how effective communication works. If we remain cognisant of the part each plays in ensuring that we are heard and understood, communication is effective and appreciation of each other's roles develops. In addition, each must exercise the ability to *listen to others* and *analyse each individual need.* Having *listened*, no effective *change* is achieved unless we *act* on the information, and *communicate* it to others.

Peers are an effective means of support, supervision and guidance yet we are often isolated in our professional practice. Stress and burnout cause ill health. We can all experience it. It is not a weakness. If we truly value one another, and wish to be effective in communication, and its rewards, we would be better placed to support, rather than knock, our colleagues. After all, it could be *you* next time!

4 Intra-disciplinary
Communicating information
Some individuals within teams withhold information. To possess information not yet available to others is often misinterpreted as *power.* Practice and service provision is only effective if information is shared. There is more *power* and *respect* gained by sharing information and resources with colleagues than from withholding it. After all, if no one knows you are holding that information – perhaps on a new treatment or approach – how can your influence and knowledge be acknowledged? Moreover, how can your colleagues improve treatment, care and interventions?

Regular professional meetings are essential to information sharing. If you are a *hoarder* by nature, this will be your opportunity to demonstrate your skill and knowledge, and at the same time, bring the rest of the team up to date.

5 Inter-disciplinary team
The admission process
Whatever your area of work, the admission or acceptance of a planned therapeutic intervention with the individual, family and/or carers is part of your role. To be effective it is essential that professional communication is coordinated. It is often the minor considerations that have an important impact on ineffective communication if omitted.

In emergency hospital admissions, other hospital and community appointments can be missed. Other professionals and agencies involved may be unaware of the admission. Even planned admissions cause communication issues. Hospital admission provokes anxiety, in even the calmest individual. People do forget to cancel appointments. Therefore, immediately after the individual is engaged in assessment it should be ascertained what other services – directly or indirectly – are involved, and what appointments may be anticipated during admission. Planned appointments that may be missed, proposed community visits and/or clinic appointments need to be noted, and each professional colleague or agency should be informed. With permission, approach the family in case they hold additional information. In addition, direct communication with individuals and agencies by the professional is essential.

It is often easier to share information relating to your involvement with an individual using a multi-copy letter. It is good practice (and will be much appreciated by other colleagues) to give the individual a copy of this letter.

The discharge process

If the needs of the individual have changed since your therapeutic intervention, it may be appropriate to arrange a joint case conference to share valuable information relating to the present and future care needs.

The individual, family and carers do feel vulnerable when intensive services are withdrawn. Even though the individual may require no immediate intervention, there is a sense of safety if it is understood that someone will be available to answer any questions they may have should a problem arise. Withdrawal of professional involvement or discharge should not take place until adequate arrangements for the continuation of essential care is agreed and in place. It is bad practice to withdraw a service or discharge the individual without adequate and effective planning. Crises can and do occur. Community services are not always easily accessible at weekends. Ten minutes of pre-withdrawal or discharge preparation will save one or more hours of crisis follow-up contact. Communication to the primary healthcare team is imperative to progress a smooth transition from hospital to home – even in rapid discharge.

It is beneficial if the individual knows the name of the community or clinic professional who is involved in their follow-on care. This is far more reassuring than being told that '*a letter will be sent to you in a week or so*'.

Avoiding unnecessary cost and time-wasting

Our lives are hectic; full of twists, turns and manoeuvres. Consequently, it is easy to become encapsulated within what *we* do – the task of daily work. It is easy to forget to inform other professionals and agencies about matters that impinge on that professionals day. If this situation is unmanaged then communication breaks down and ill feeling and rivalry ensues. When one is busy, time is of the essence – it is precious and valued. Visiting the individual at home, only to find that the visit has clashed with an unknown clinic appointment leaves the professional feeling frustrated and angry, as if time has been stolen.

For those arguing that this is additional bureaucracy gone mad, the above guidance, if acted on, and carefully followed, is cheaper than the cost of a missed appointment or confusion arising from poor communication. A wasted community visit, or the loss of money due to a missed benefits agency appointment far outweigh the cost involved in effective communication between busy professionals and agencies.

What can I do to improve personal communication?

Common sense, courtesy and good manners form the basis of effective communication. Allow for a great deal of personal effort, patience, practice and disappointment, but do prevail. We all have an individual responsibility to improve communication. Think: *what would I like from others? ME* is the *master key*. It *is* possible for an individual, and team, to effectively improve communication.

6 Middle management

Communicating change

The middle manager plays a pivotal role in the communication of change. Change in any organisation is unsettling. Half-truth and rumours need little encouragement for dissemination and cause dissatisfaction. It is easier to have all your colleagues on board the ship than it is to stop the ship, circle, and collect those who have fallen overboard. Change affects all members of the intra-disciplinary team; this in turn impacts on the inter-disciplinary team and *ultimately individualised care*. To share, and be fully conversant with the change and the process involved, can and does lead to team support. Involvement and a sense of being part of the change process, rather than excluded and unworthy of consideration, are essential for effective communication and ownership of change.

7 Senior management

Senior and middle managers need to know the detail of the job each employee undertakes. It is not essential for the manager to be from the same discipline but it is necessary for him/her to be familiar with the exact role of the employee. Only then can respect, mutual understanding and communication be effective. Similarly, the manager needs to share with the employee what his/her own role entails.

One can communicate with a colleague and still encounter misunderstanding. Anyone with a teenage son or daughter will know that even when the benefits of having a clean, tidy room have been explained – for the hundredth time – and a check has been made to ensure understanding of the guidance, numerous reminders administered, and the consequences of lack of action explained, the room remains unclean. Each professional can only try to improve communication – to make communication clear and unambiguous. Human nature dictates that some communications will go unheeded or misinterpreted. However, we are not challenging teenagers – we are adults who would like a good working environment.

Setting the example

During times of pressure and stress, effective communication is the first thing to suffer, yet it reduces pressure and stress. Effective communication frees time to deal with other matters that are important to individualised care. Effective communication comes from the top. Senior managers lead by example: only then will the employee find the tasks that he/she is set easier to work with and control. However, a lack of such leadership is not an excuse for one's actions, inactions or omissions.

Direction on effective communication comes from senior managers. If the directive is clear, emphasising that effective communication is important, then it is likely that the practice will disseminate throughout the organisation. However, there is little benefit issuing directives if, in personal practice, the manager does not lead by example.

The personal touch

Emails and memos have made life easier for the busy manager. The increasing lack of pleasantries within the communication and the formal directness and abbreviation means that it is hard to perceive the *literal intention* of the message we receive. Managers should be aware of this change and make written communication accessible. Time to include the pleasantries should be spent when developing the communication. Avoid misinterpretation.

Breaking bad news

Never, communicate bad news in writing. This should always be undertaken personally. If you wish to speak to someone about an issue, this should be undertaken immediately. It is poor and ineffective communication to leave an employee waiting overnight or over a weekend wondering if there is a problem. If the matter involves discipline or reprimand, wait until you are able to see the person. If you have to send a written communication, include information about the anticipated nature of the topic. Likewise, if the meeting is set up verbally, involving a routine matter, and is to take place in a few days, give some indication as to the topic. This avoids rumour, speculation and anxiety. After all, a happy workforce is more effective than an unhappy one. Moreover, they are willing to give in excess of their hours to the organisation – so why disrupt it!

We have ascertained that personal face-to-face communication is far more productive in terms of the manager–employee relationship. It cannot be overemphasised that if the employee you wish to speak to is in the next room or same building and is immediately available – stand up – walk out the door and *speak to him or her*. This will be better received than an email or memo from someone who is only feet away. *It establishes and earns respect.*

Communicating with a colleague

It is frustrating to feel that ones professional communications and the important issues you wish to raise within and outwith the team at junior, peer, intra-disciplinary, inter-disciplinary, middle and senior management are disregarded, unheard or dismissed. It is essential to remember that effective communication is a two-way process. Often information needs reinforcement and clarification. All parties need to understand what is:
➤ required of them
➤ said
➤ not said.

To keep interaction effective, and the inevitable knock-on effect on the individual, family/carers interventions, running smoothly. Do:

- ➤ write
- ➤ meet personally
- ➤ telephone
- ➤ email
- ➤ fax
- ➤ thank colleagues
- ➤ respect colleagues
- ➤ acknowledge your limitations
- ➤ seek help when needed
- ➤ understand the demands on others
- ➤ be aware of others feelings
- ➤ assume that you need to clarify your actions
- ➤ keep communicating effectively – even if others give up.

This is basic good manners; sadly, it is often forgotten!

CONCLUSION

> Some people feel that what we do is easy . . . straightforward . . . but it isn't easy and straightforward for the individual and family . . . we have to help them untangle the web of dis-ease they find themselves facing . . .
> (A community psychiatric nurse in clinical supervision.)

This chapter reflects on a small number of examples of poor and *effective* communication. There is probably an almanac of ineffective communication examples that one could describe: each one of us having our own personal story! It is intended to demonstrate that, with a little work from *you*, as an integral individual, effective communication can happen within and outwith *your* organisation: *you* just have to give it brain space and effort. It is not a *thing* to do later but an instrument to use constantly – always at the forefront of everyday activities.

Effective communication is cost-effective and saves time. Misunderstanding, anger, frustration, complaints and worry – *for the individual, family and carer, other professionals and oneself* – can be avoided provided we communicate effectively.

Why keep walking into doors? Life is difficult enough! Each individual within and across an organisation has a responsibility to communicate effectively – not just for oneself but for others whose lives we touch in one way or another and who are unable to care directly or indirectly for themselves. Effective communication is the master key . . . it fits all locks and opens the way to therapeutic treatment and interventions.[1]

Having cited all of the above, none of this holds any importance if the receiver of communication does not *listen*. This *two-way process* is imperative if communication is to be effective.

No professional wants the individual, family or carers to suffer as a consequence of his or her inaction – yet we risk this every day through poor communication. It is not *their* responsibility – it is *our* responsibility to make communication effective and meaningful to the best of our ability and understanding. If there were just seven words of wisdom in professional practice and effective communication these would be:

Never assume people know . . . they do not!

POST-READING EXERCISE 12.1

Time: 30 minutes

Reconsider the Pre-reading exercise 12.1

- What changes, identified in question 1, would you now make to improve communication in your answers to question 2?
- Has your list changed?
- If yes, how?

ACKNOWLEDGEMENT

© Cooper J. *Stepping into Palliative Care 1: relationships and responses.* 2nd ed. Oxford: Radcliffe Publishing; 2006. Reproduced with the permission of the copyright holder. I am grateful to Jo Cooper for allowing me to reproduce an edited version of my chapter in this book. Thank you.

REFERENCES

1 Cooper DB. The standard guide to . . . communication. *Nurs Stand.* 1994; **8**(29): 42–3.
2 McLeod WT, managing editor. *Collins Dictionary and Thesaurus*: in one volume. Glasgow: HarperCollins; 1991.
3 Cambridge Dictionary online. Available at: http://dictionary.cambridge.org/

CHAPTER 13

Spirituality, mental health–substance use

Christopher CH Cook

PRE-READING EXERCISE 13.1

Time: 30 minutes
- What is spirituality?
- How is this different, or is it, from religion?

INTRODUCTION

Spirituality is an increasingly important topic in healthcare. A growing evidence base suggests that spirituality and religion are protective factors that reduce the risk of a wide range of physical and mental disorders. They also influence use of medical services and outcome following treatment. Furthermore, individuals wish spirituality and religion to be taken into account in the planning and delivery of the care that they receive.[1-3] It would therefore seem that there is a good prima facie case for making spiritual care routinely available as a component of healthcare provision. However, spirituality and religion are also proving to be controversial topics in healthcare. In the UK in 2009, a nurse was suspended (albeit later reinstated) for offering to pray for an ill person.[4] In 2008, in the journal *Psychiatric Bulletin*, heated correspondence followed an editorial in which it was suggested that spirituality and religion should be taken into account in the assessment and treatment of mental disorder.[5-8] It would therefore seem that spiritual care is a subject of disagreement among healthcare professionals.

Within the wider world of healthcare, and alongside specialities such as palliative care, mental health and substance use are among those fields in which spirituality and religion have attracted particular attention. This should not be surprising, for they are concerned with some of the most deeply held human beliefs and values. At a purely psychological level we might therefore expect that disorders of affect, cognition and behaviour might have some impact upon spiritual and religious belief, and conversely, that such beliefs would be likely to have an impact upon the expression of psychiatric disorder.

What, then, is the nature of the inter-relationships between spirituality, religion, mental disorder and substance use, and how might these relationships influence assessment, treatment and service provision? Before attempting to provide some answers to these questions, it is necessary to consider the nature and concept of spirituality.

Spirituality

Spirituality is a difficult term to define.[9,10] It is undoubtedly capable of diverse and, at times, mutually contradictory definitions. Thus, for example, in the minds of some it is intimately related to the concept of religion, whereas for others it is the very antithesis of religion. However, generally speaking, it tends to assume a more individual, subjective and personal quality than does religion. Whereas it is self-evident that not all people are religious, it is arguable that all human beings are spiritual. It is therefore possible to be spiritual, but not religious. Some people would argue that it is also possible to be religious but not spiritual, and still others would argue that they are neither spiritual nor religious. However, if spirituality is concerned with relationships, with deeply held values and beliefs, and with meaning and purpose in life, it is difficult to see how it is possible for a person not to be spiritual unless they have nothing and no one that matters to them.

There are many definitions of spirituality, and this is not the place to assess their relative merits. However, the following is offered as an example of a more inclusive approach:

> *Spirituality is a distinctive, potentially creative and universal dimension of human experience arising both within the inner subjective awareness of individuals and within communities, social groups and traditions. It may be experienced as relationship with that which is intimately 'inner', immanent and personal, within the self and others, and/or as relationship with that which is wholly 'other', transcendent and beyond the self. It is experienced as being of fundamental or ultimate importance and is thus concerned with matters of meaning and purpose in life, truth and values.*[9]

In passing, it is important to note that religion is also a difficult concept to define, but that it is usually understood in terms of socially shared beliefs, behaviours, traditions and experiences. In research terms, it is easier to measure as it involves easily observable functions (often referred to as 'religiosity') such as attendance at religious services or involvement in personal religious devotions, or self-identified affiliation to a particular community or faith tradition. However, it also has its subjective aspects and it is difficult to see how religion can be completely devoid of spirituality unless certain negative patterns (e.g. discrepancies of moral behaviour) are redefined (usually according to someone else's values), as being a lack of spirituality rather than as a negative manifestation of a particular form of spirituality.

Both spirituality and religion are important in the healthcare context. It is therefore important to be able to enquire about both in a sensitive fashion. When the individual, family or carers identify themselves as belonging to a particular faith tradition, assumptions should not be made about what that might mean. The significance and expression of this self-identified religious belonging needs further exploration in order to understand exactly what it means to *this* person, rather than to any notion of orthodoxy or to members of that religion in general. Similarly, self-identification as 'not spiritual' or 'not religious' still leaves important scope for enquiry about relationships, value, purpose and meaning in life.

MENTAL HEALTH

Mental health is also notoriously difficult to define. The World Health Organization definition of mental health does not include any explicit reference to spirituality:

> Mental health is defined as a state of well-being in which every individual realizes his or her own potential, can cope with the normal stresses of life, can work productively and fruitfully, and is able to make a contribution to her or his community.[11]

However, health and 'well-being' are concepts that invite reflection upon spiritual as well as physical, social and psychological aspects of what it means to be a flourishing human being. Because spirituality is concerned with such issues as relationship, value, meaning and purpose it is also very difficult (if not impossible) to separate from the kinds of issues that arise when thought, mood, perception or behaviour are disordered as a result of mental illness. Spiritual issues therefore, not surprisingly, arise in most clinical areas of psychiatric practice.[12]

Statistically, religious involvement is associated with a greater sense of well-being, more positive mood states, greater satisfaction with life, better psychological coping and better mental health (*see* review by Koenig, pp. 43–81).[13] However, in a minority of studies it is associated with worse mental health, and in some cases it is associated with negative emotional traits (pp. 70–81).[13] There are also clearly forms of 'pathological spirituality', such as those associated with some cults, which are especially associated with psychiatric morbidity.[14]

In the case of major psychiatric disorders, such as schizophrenia or bipolar affective disorder, the evidence of a protective effect of spirituality or religion is largely lacking. However, there is also a dearth of research in this area, and therefore little is known with confidence about the nature of the relationship.[13,15] Furthermore, the relationship between psychosis and spirituality is a complex one, within which mental and spiritual experiences become closely intertwined. The need for sensitive and compassionate spiritual care of those who experience such problems is great.[16]

Koenig identifies 10 ways in which religious beliefs or practices may improve mental health, which might reasonably be understood to apply to spirituality.[10,13] They may:

- promote a positive world view
- help to make sense of difficult situations
- give purpose and meaning
- discourage maladaptive coping
- enhance social support
- promote 'other-directedness'
- help to release the need for control

➤ provide and encourage forgiveness
➤ encourage thankfulness
➤ provide hope.

Spirituality and religiosity may also be incorporated into treatment. Options include specifically religious approaches to psychotherapy, and utilisation of the social support available in faith communities. However, Koenig,[13] also warns of the dangers and limitations of such approaches. Mental health professionals often have little training or competency in such work, and discrepancies between the spiritual or religious world view of the professional and individual can lead to ethical problems or complexities of transference and counter-transference.[13]

SUBSTANCE USE

The relationship between religion and substance use is well demonstrated by research, especially among groups of young people. Numerous studies have shown that affiliation with a faith community is a protective factor that reduces the likelihood of use of illicit substances or excessive use of socially sanctioned substances, such as alcohol or nicotine.[17] There are various possible mechanisms, by which this protective effect may operate.

1 Moral teaching provided within faith communities may operate directly to discourage substance use.
2 Belonging to a peer group that does not use substances (and/or does not use them excessively) may provide a form of modelling that encourages conforming behaviour amongst those who wish to belong to the group.
3 The social support provided by a faith community may enable alternative coping mechanisms that reduce the need to use substances as a means of coping with stress.
4 The better mental health, or more positive mood, enabled by membership of a faith community may reduce the need for use of substances as a coping mechanism.

It might be imagined that the chances of being offered drugs (especially illicit drugs) are less for those who belong to faith communities. However, although there is some evidence for this, the magnitude of difference is small and does not appear to explain the difference in prevalence of substance use.[18]

By way of example, one study of 7666 church-affiliated young people in the UK in 1995, showed that 23% of those aged between 12 and 16 years had been offered illicit drugs, but only 10% had tried them. (Comparable figures for those aged 17 to 30 years were 46% and 23% [18]). Church attendance, agreement with a statement of Christian belief, and personal spiritual practices (bible reading and prayer) were associated with a lesser likelihood of having tried drugs (and also of having smoked cigarettes or drunk alcohol). However, church attendance appeared to be a more important factor in the younger group and personal spiritual practices were more important among the older young people, perhaps reflecting a shift during adolescence towards personal spirituality as a more important protective influence.[19]

SUBSTANCE USE PROBLEMS

Our understanding of the relationship between spirituality and substance use problems has been influenced by various historical factors concerned with the relationship between religion and excessive alcohol consumption (or in the case of Islam, any alcohol consumption). During the 20th century it has also been profoundly influenced by the emergence of Alcoholics Anonymous (AA) and its sister organisations as a significant resource in support of recovery.[20,21] Arguably, there is an intrinsic relationship between substance dependence and spirituality, in that the former is inherently a spiritual problem by virtue of the way in which it impacts upon relationships, values and purpose in life. However, the influence of Alcoholics Anonymous and other '12-Step'[22] programmes, which affirm a spiritual rather than religious approach to recovery, has been enormous and this has probably done most in drawing attention to the need to address the spiritual dimension of problems associated with substance dependence.

The spirituality enshrined in Alcoholics Anonymous principles draws on the Christian tradition, but is importantly modified through a psychological and medical perspective influenced by William James, a pioneer in the study of the psychology of religion.[17] James' influence is particularly evident in the reference to 'God as we understood Him', and in the stripping out of any traditional religious, theological or doctrinal formulations. The emphasis is rather upon the recognition of one's own 'powerlessness', a turning towards a transcendent source of help, and the recognition of a moral frame of reference. It is also important to note that Step 12 provides an emphasis on helping others. This is not 'self-help', but rather 'mutual-help'.

This mutual-help programme has since been applied to those experiencing problems using other substances, as well as to a variety of non-substance-based patterns of behaviour that might be considered forms of 'addiction', (e.g. gambling, sexual behaviour and eating disorders). It has also influenced professionally led treatment programmes for substance use problems.[23,24]

Other approaches to the treatment of substance use problems within which spirituality has been emphasised have included a variety of religiously based programmes, where a programme of recovery is devised that includes prayer, study of scripture, meditation or other religious devotions. Obviously, such programmes are primarily, but not exclusively, of interest to those who enter treatment with an affiliation to (or at least a sympathy for) a particular religious tradition. It is also possible to introduce spirituality as a component of a comprehensive treatment approach in a broad way, so as to address the needs of those who come from any of the world's major faith traditions or none of them.[25] What would seem to be important is the recognition of the spiritual needs of people recovering from substance use problems, and a sensitivity to providing an accessible way to address these needs during the course of treatment. That might be provided by involvement in a 12-step programme, or through chaplaincy support, or through an explicitly religious ethos. However, the research evidence that is beginning to emerge from this field does suggest that it is beneficial to good outcomes to address the spiritual needs of such people in some way.[17]

MENTAL HEALTH–SUBSTANCE USE

We know, then, that spirituality exerts a protective effect against both mental health and substance use problems. In each case, there are multiple possible mechanisms. However, spirituality is also probably best understood as a multi dimensional concept.[26] Which aspects of spirituality exert the protective effect in each case? At present little empirical evidence exists upon which to base an answer to this question, but there is reason to believe that different aspects of spirituality may reduce the risk of mental health–substance use problems.

In a study of 2621 twins on the Virginia twin registry, it was found to be impossible to separate spirituality from religiosity in a factor analysis.[27] However, the authors found that different dimensions of religiosity were associated with reduced risk of mental disorders (depression, anxiety disorders and bulimia) and various categories of substance use problems. Two dimensions of religiosity, specifically social religiosity and thankfulness, were associated with reduced risk of mental health–substance use problems. Four dimensions of religiosity (general religiosity, belief in a God involved in human affairs, forgiveness and belief in a judgemental God) were associated with reduced risk of substance use problems (and adult antisocial behaviour) only. Only one dimension of religiosity, an attitude of 'un-vengefulness', was predictive of reduced risk for mental health problems only.

Given the benefits in treatment of both mental health and substance use problems, we would expect that spirituality would have benefits in the treatment of individuals experiencing mental health–substance use problems. Research is beginning to provide evidence in support of this expectation.

In a study in Washington, DC, of 27 women with histories of physical or sexual abuse and mental health–substance use problems, spirituality was identified by participants as an important influence sustaining recovery.[28] In another study, people experiencing mental health–substance use problems at a specialist unit in New York reported that they viewed spirituality as 'essential to their recovery'. Nurses in the same unit, while being similarly spiritually orientated as the individuals, underestimated the extent to which individuals considered this to be an important factor in their treatment.[29] Medical students at the same unit were significantly less spiritually orientated and did not consider spirituality to be an important factor in treatment.[30]

There is evidence to support the contention that paying attention to spiritual factors in treatment improves substance-related outcomes for people experiencing mental health–substance use problems.[31] In a study of homeless veterans experiencing mental health–substance use problems, it was found that spiritual well-being was one of a number of 'transforming experiences' that reduced readmission rates.[32] Moreover, there appears to be particular evidence of the benefits of religious coping among women trauma survivors experiencing mental health–substance use problems.[33] However, even if it is usually a beneficial factor, spirituality (or at least religiosity) is a variable that can work both ways.

In a study in Switzerland of 115 people with non-affective psychotic illness[34,35] (among which, 23% had mental health–substance use problems, rising to 63% where nicotine dependence was included), religious involvement was significantly inversely correlated to substance use. Religious coping was found to:

➤ reduce substance use in 14% and increase it in 3%
➤ lessen psychotic and other symptoms in 54%, but increase such symptoms in 10%
➤ increase social integration in 28%, but increase social isolation in 3%
➤ reduce the risk of suicide attempts in 33%, but increase the risk in 10%
➤ improve adherence to psychiatric treatment in 16%, but result in opposition to such treatment in 15%.

While the overall benefits of religious involvement and religious coping are evident, it is important to recognise that the relationship can work both ways. Sometimes, religiosity (and presumably also spirituality) may make things worse.

Twelve-step groups have been established that are particularly orientated towards the needs of people with mental health–substance use problems. There is some research evidence that attendance at these groups is associated with better adherence to medication, lower symptom severity at one year follow-up, and reduced likelihood of readmission during the same follow-up period.[36,37]

GOOD PRACTICE

The need to undertake an assessment of spiritual need should not now be controversial. Not only does evidence suggest that spirituality is relevant to healthcare outcomes, but individuals indicate that they wish their spiritual needs to be addressed in treatment. A spiritual needs assessment is simply good practice, and an example of such good practice is commended in the Department of Health guide *Religion or Belief* (pp. 33–4).[38] There are many ways, in which, such assessments may be undertaken,[39] and they do not need to be time consuming. For example, a system based on four short screening questions, using the acronym 'FICAA' has been suggested:[40]

➤ What is your **F**aith tradition?
➤ How **I**mportant is your faith to you?
➤ What is your **C**hurch or community of faith?
➤ How do your religious and spiritual beliefs **A**pply to your health?
➤ How might we **A**ddress your spiritual needs?

Clearly, such assessment should be conducted professionally and within an ethical framework that does not allow proselytising or discrimination. The American Psychiatric Association have published guidelines, within which, the undertaking of a spiritual and religious assessment is understood as a part of the maintaining of respect for peoples' beliefs, and within which, the imposing of psychiatrists' beliefs on the individual (whether those beliefs be religious, antireligious or ideologic), is explicitly proscribed.[41]

CONCLUSION

Spirituality and religiosity are important factors to be considered in understanding the aetiology and proper treatment of mental health–substance use problems. Where such problems co-occur there is double reason to take these factors seriously. Good practice should, at least, involve a proper assessment of spiritual needs.

There is also evidence to suggest that incorporation of spirituality into treatment is associated with good outcomes. This need not mean that treatment programmes must be explicitly religious, although some are. Professional treatment programmes and mutual help groups incorporating a secular or pluralist approach to spirituality, such as that espoused by AA and its sister organisations, are also effective.

POST-READING EXERCISE 13.2

Time: 30 minutes
- What is spirituality?
- How is this different, or is it, from religion?
- How would you ask the question around religion and spirituality? Consider your own feelings in understanding self.

REFERENCES

1 Koenig HG. *Spirituality in Patient Care.* 2nd ed. Philadelphia, PA: Templeton Foundation Press; 2007.
2 Koenig HG. *Medicine, Religion and Health: where science and spirituality meet.* West Conshohocken, PA: Templeton Foundation Press; 2008.
3 Koenig HG, McCullough ME, Larson DB. *Handbook of Religion and Health.* New York: Oxford University Press; 2001.
4 Wilkes D, Sears N. *Prosecuted for Praying: nurse who faces sack after offering to pray for sick patient.* 2009. Available at: www.dailymail.co.uk/news/article-1133423/Nurse-faces-sack-offering-pray-sick-patient.html (accessed 9 June 2010), and Gledhill R. *Victory for Suspended Christian Nurse.* 2009. www.timesonline.co.uk/tol/comment/faith/article5675452.ece (accessed 9 June 2010).
5 Koenig HG. Religion and mental health: what should psychiatrists do? *Psychiatr Bull.* 2008; **32**: 201–3.
6 Poole R, Higgo R, Strong G, *et al.* Religion, psychiatry and professional boundaries. *Psychiatr Bull.* [Letter]. 2008; **32**: 356–7.
7 Lepping P. Religion, psychiatry and professional boundaries. *Psychiatr Bull.* [Letter]. 2008; **32**: 357.
8 Mushtaq I, Hafeez MA. Psychiatrists and role of religion in mental health. *Psychiatr Bull.* [Letter]. 2008; **32**: 395.
9 Cook CCH. Addiction and spirituality. *Addiction.* 2004; **99**: 539–51.
10 Sims A, Cook CCH. Spirituality in Psychiatry. In: Cook C, Powell A, Sims A, editors. *Spirituality and Psychiatry.* London: Royal College of Psychiatrists Press; 2009. pp. 1–15.
11 World Health Organization. *Mental Health: a state of wellbeing.* Available at: www.who.int/features/factfiles/mental_health/en/index.html (accessed 9 June 2010).
12 Cook C, Powell A, Sims A, editors. *Spirituality and Psychiatry.* London: Royal College of Psychiatrists Press; 2009.
13 Koenig HG. *Faith and Mental Health.* Philadelphia, PA: Templeton Foundation Press; 2005.
14 Crowley N, Jenkinson G. Pathological spirituality. In: Cook C, Powell A, Sims A, editors. *Spirituality and Psychiatry.* London: Royal College of Psychiatrists Press; 2009. pp. 254–72.

15 Chamberlain TJ, Hall CA. *Realized Religion*. Philadelphia, PA: Templeton Foundation Press; 2000.

16 Mitchell S, Roberts G. Psychosis. In: Cook C, Powell A, Sims A, editors. *Spirituality and Psychiatry*. London: Royal College of Psychiatrists Press; 2009. pp. 39–60.

17 Cook CCH. Substance misuse. In: Cook C, Powell A, Sims A, editors. *Spirituality and Psychiatry*. London: Royal College of Psychiatrists Press; 2009. pp. 139–68.

18 Cook CCH, Goddard D, Westall R. Knowledge and experience of drug use amongst church affiliated young people. *Drug Alcohol Depend.* 1997; **46**: 9–17.

19 Hope LC, Cook CCH. The role of Christian commitment in predicting drug use amongst church affiliated young people. *Mental Health, Religion & Culture.* 2001; **4**: 109–17.

20 Cook CCH. *Alcohol, Addiction and Christian Ethics*. Cambridge: Cambridge University Press; 2006.

21 Cook CCH. AA's first European experience and the spiritual experience of AA. *Addiction.* 2007; **102**: 846–7.

22 Alcoholics Anonymous. *Twelve Steps and Twelve Traditions*. New York: Alcoholics Anonymous World Services; 1977.

23 Cook CCH. The Minnesota model in the management of drug and alcohol dependency: miracle method or myth? Part I. The philosophy and the programme. *Br J Addict.* 1988; **83**: 625–34.

24 Cook CCH. The Minnesota model in the management of drug and alcohol dependency: miracle method or myth? Part II. Evidence and conclusions. *Br J Addict.* 1988; **83**: 735–48.

25 Jackson P, Cook CCH. Introduction of a spirituality group in a community service for people with drinking problems. *J Subst Use.* 2005; **10**: 375–83.

26 Fetzer I, National Institute on Aging Working Group. *Multidimensional Measurement of Religiousness/Spirituality for Use in Health Research*. Kalamazoo, MI: Fetzer Institute; 1999.

27 Kendler KS, Liu X-Q, Gardner CO, *et al.* Dimensions of religiosity and their relationship to lifetime psychiatric and substance use disorders. *Am J Psychiatry.* 2003; **160**: 496–503.

28 Harris M, Fallot RD, Berley RW. Qualitative interviews on substance abuse relapse and prevention among female trauma survivors. *Psychiatr Serv.* 2005; **56**: 1292–6.

29 McDowell D, Galanter M, Goldfarb L, *et al.* Spirituality and the treatment of the dually diagnosed: an investigation of patient and staff attitudes. *J Addict Dis.* 1996; **15**: 55–68.

30 Goldfarb LM, Galanter M, McDowell D, *et al.* Medical student and patient attitudes toward religion and spirituality in the recovery process. *Am J Drug Alcohol Abuse.* 1996; **22**: 549–61.

31 Davis KE, O'Neill SJ. A focus group analysis of relapse prevention strategies for persons with substance use and mental disorders. *Psychiatr Serv.* 2005; **56**: 1288–91.

32 Benda BB. Life-course theory of readmission of substance abusers among homeless veterans. *Psychiatr Serv.* 2004; **55**: 1308–10.

33 Fallot RD, Heckman JP. Religious/spiritual coping among women trauma survivors with mental health and substance use disorders. *J Behav Health Serv Res.* 2005; **32**: 215–26.

34 Mohr S, Brandt P-Y, Borras L, *et al.* Toward an integration of spirituality and religiousness into the psychosocial dimension of schizophrenia. *Am J Psychiatry.* 163: 1952–9.

35 Huguelet P, Borras L, Gilliéron C, *et al.* Influence of spirituality and religiousness on substance misuse in patients with schizophrenia or schizo-affective disorder. *Subst Use Misuse.* 2009; **44**: 502–13.

36 Magura S, Laudet AB, Mahmood D, *et al.* Adherence to medication regimens and participation in dual-focus self-help groups. *Psychiatr Serv.* 2002; **53**: 310–16.

37 Magura S, Knight EL, Vogel HS, *et al.* Mediators of effectiveness in dual-focus self-help groups. *Am J Drug Alcohol Abuse.* 2003; **29**: 301–22.

38 Department of Health. *Religion or Belief: a practical guide for the NHS.* London: Department of Health; 2009. Available at: www.suffolk.nhs.uk/LinkClick.aspx?fileticket=AOdBpto%2B DkQ%3D&tabid=1439&mid=2879 (accessed 9 June 2010).

39 Culliford L, Eagger S. Assessing spiritual needs. In: Cook C, Powell A, Sims A, editors. *Spirituality and Psychiatry.* London: Royal College of Psychiatrists Press; 2009. pp. 16–38.

40 Puchalski CM, Roma AL. Taking a spiritual history allows clinicians to understand patients more fully. *J Palliat Med.* 2000; **3**: 129–37.

41 Committee on Religion and Psychiatry. Guidelines regarding possible conflict between psychiatrists' religious commitments and psychiatric practice. *Am J Psychiatry.* 1990; **147**: 542.

TO LEARN MORE

- Spirituality and Psychiatry Special Interest Group of the Royal College of Psychiatrists: www.rcpsych.ac.uk/college/specialinterestgroups/spirituality.aspx
- Mental Health Foundation: www.mentalhealth.org.uk/information/mental-health-a-z/spirituality/
- Project for Spirituality, Theology and Health, Durham University, UK: www.dur.ac.uk/spirituality.health/
- Centre for Spirituality, Theology and Health, Duke University, USA: www.spiritualityand health.duke.edu/
- Alcoholics Anonymous: www.alcoholics-anonymous.org.uk/
- Dual Recovery Anonymous: www.draonline.org/

CHAPTER 14

Sexuality, mental health–substance use

Lyn Matthews and Jon Hibberd

PRE-READING EXERCISE 14.1

Time: 10 minutes
Before reading this chapter, reflect on your understanding of sexuality.
- What impact does it have upon you?
- How do you see it expressed?
- Are you comfortable in raising the subject?

INTRODUCTION

At the outset, this chapter refers to the concept of sexuality in its broadest terms. It then looks at the Armistead Centre, identifying the needs of the lesbian, homosexual, bisexual and transgender communities. The first part of this chapter is adapted from the field of palliative care, who lead the way in dissemination of knowledge and understanding around sexuality.

DEFINING SEXUALITY

Numerous attempts have been made to define sexuality with differing emphasis placed on its social, psychological, spiritual and physical attributes. The fact so many definitions exist suggests that as an integral component of who each person is, it is unique. Sexuality is primary to our self-understanding and social role but it is also a private, hidden aspect of ourselves that we may choose, or not choose, to share with others.[1]

Sexuality comes into all aspects of existence, involving biological and social aspects of the body. It is complex and contextual.[2]

If the definitions are placed within the context of mental health–substance use, their importance becomes vital in the care of the individual experiencing mental health–substance use problems. Such conditions have a significant physical, psychological, emotional, social and spiritual effect upon all aspects of a person's sexuality. In all its diversity, it is inevitably affected.

SELF-ASSESSMENT EXERCISE 14.1

> **Time: 15 minutes**
> For someone experiencing mental health–substance use problems, how do you think his or her sexuality will be affected?
> *Try to group your thoughts into headings, for example:*
> - *physical* – change in body image and health
> - *emotional* – anxiety, fear, low self-esteem and anger
> - *social* – touch, communication and impact on work
> - *spiritual* – challenge to faith. Finding a spiritual faith/path.

When answering the self-assessment question you will have identified many examples that illustrate clearly how important sexuality is in our lives. It is fundamental to the way people:
➤ share intimacy
➤ experience physical closeness
➤ view themselves
➤ are perceived by others.

Sexuality and body image are closely linked with roles and relationships within families, at work and in society.[3] It includes, but should never be limited to, sexual intercourse and sexual function.

EXPRESSING SEXUALITY

A way of looking at sexuality is demonstrated in the Sexuality Flower Model (Figure 14.1).

SELF-ASSESSMENT EXERCISE 14.2

> **Time: 5 minutes**
> Look at the Sexuality Flower Model (Figure 14.1 opposite), then reflect on:
> - what you have done today
> - the emotions and feelings you have experienced
> - the communication you have had with adults, children; even animals.

You should be able to identify many words in the Sexuality Flower Model that would describe what you have experienced. Possibly, several words would describe your experience, embracing an action accompanied by an emotion, or feeling. *This is your unique, personal expression of sexuality.*

ADDRESSING THE 'TABOO'

Until now, the focus has been about raising awareness of the influence of sexuality. This section takes a different approach in attempting to dispel the fears that many

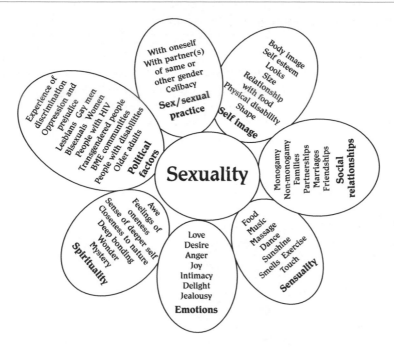

These all add up to how we define ourselves as sexual beings
Sexuality = sexual selfhood
Sexuality involves our relationships with ourselves, those around us
and the society in which we live – whether we identify as gay,
heterosexual, lesbian, bisexual, transgender, or celibate

FIGURE 14.1 Sexuality Flower Model
Permission was kindly given to use the Sexuality Flower Model by the Centre for HIV and
Sexual Health, 22 Collegiate Crescent, Sheffield, S10 2BA. Model originally devised by Carol
Painter and Jo Adams, and used in the training manual on sexuality: 'Explore, Dream, Discover'
(2004). For more information, telephone: 01142 261900 or email: admin@chiv.nhs.uk.

professionals have in addressing the subject of sexuality with the individual and
family.

The main difficulty that professionals experience is *'I don't know what to say'*. This
can be for many reasons, which we will touch upon later. Sexuality exists separately
from sexual function.[4] Often, the two terms are used synonymously. However,
confusion often arises because they are different aspects of the same complex of
emotions and behaviours.

SELF-ASSESSMENT EXERCISE 14.3

Time: 5 minutes
- *Think* – about your understanding of the difference between sexuality and
  sexual function.
- *Reflect* – on these issues and their impact on you.

People may wish to talk about the difficulties they are experiencing with their sexuality or sexual function. However, they may not know *how* to talk about it or *who* to talk to. It is important not to assume that the individual, who does not initiate discussion, does not have concerns about sexuality. People often *'suffer in silence'* because they assume that if sexuality and intimacy were important, professionals would discuss them.[5]

As professionals (and individuals ourselves), we have our own unique set of beliefs, attitudes and values. These influence whether we perceive issues of sexuality to be an integral part of care.

SELF-ASSESSMENT EXERCISE 14.4

Time: 20 minutes

This exercise is challenging. Listed are reasons why professionals feel unable to address sexuality.

1 *Reflect on these.*
2 *Which influences your approach?*
   - I don't know what to say.
   - I don't think sexuality is an issue for people experiencing mental health–substance use problems.
   - My religious belief inhibits me from talking of such things.
   - I need special training to talk about something so personal.
   - I would feel very embarrassed about talking about it.
   - It just never enters my mind to talk about it.
   - That's someone else's job to deal with that sort of thing.
   - I think it's a vital part of care. I do address the issue of sexuality.

It could be that you did not identify with any of the comments in the self-assessment exercise (14.4). Professionals still need to learn about:

➤ the professional use of self
➤ having a high level of self-knowledge
➤ the uniqueness and value of others.[6]

SELF-ASSESSMENT EXERCISE 14.5

Time: 5 minutes

Look at the Sexuality Flower Model (Figure 14.1, p.183).
   - How well do you know yourself?

Being comfortable with one's sexual identity, and all that embraces is important when working with the individual. Professionals have a key role to play in helping the individual and family resolve difficulties they may be experiencing with their sexuality.

EXAMPLES OF BEST PRACTICE
Before reading on, reflect on the following seven points[7,8]
This list was devised as pre-requisites for addressing needs relating to the individuals sexuality.

1 **Assessment and timing** – ongoing assessment and appropriate timing of discussion.
2 **Self-awareness of the interviewer** – acknowledge own prejudice and bias. Be willing and able to put these to one side.
3 **Privacy** – setting and timing.
4 **Confidentiality** – acknowledge confidentiality with the individual.
5 **Permission giving** – gain the individuals permission to talk – or not.
6 **Language** – use appropriate language.
7 **Boundaries** – set time boundaries for self and the individual.

Problems with sexuality and sexual function can often have a 'spin off' effect, for example exacerbating feelings of low self-esteem and low self-worth. These feelings, if not addressed, may cause difficulties in relationship that assume greater magnitude than they are.

Each situation you encounter will be different. Therefore, it is important to remember the five basic principles that hold true for any situation.

1 Active listening.
2 Reflecting back to check thoughts and feelings.
3 Be empathic.
4 Do not judge.
5 Be self-aware.

The four misconceptions held are:

1 **Age** – do not assume that sexuality and sexual function is no longer important to older individuals.
2 **Heterosexuality** – do not ignore the possibility of homosexual/lesbian relationships.
3 **Being single** – do not assume that sexuality and sexual function is not an issue for people not in a relationship.
4 **Mental health–substance use care status** – do not assume that the individual has no interest in sexual activity.

ARMISTEAD CENTRE: A PROFESSIONAL'S PERCEPTION
It is easy when one lives within the suggested social 'norms' of society to take 'who we are' for granted. It is quite easy to ignore and forget those who live on societies margins, such as people who use substances and the mentally ill. Often, some of the most vulnerable people of society fall through the net, or are failed by those who are supposed to help them. When services are set up, they need to be inclusive – to all. However, certain groups whose religion, race, colour, or sexual orientation deviates from these 'norms', find it difficult to access health and social care services.

Often the individual from a diverse group will address the problems within her/his own community and develop services from grassroots level. The Armistead

Centre[9] is one such project that was set up to address the sexual health needs of homosexual and bisexual men. Established in 1997, the project has gone on to develop services that are inclusive to all from the lesbian, homosexual, bisexual and transgender communities and takes a holistic and evidence-based approach to diverse needs. The project is one of the few projects in the UK that provides substance use professionals with support, and outreach programmes aimed at working with individuals directly in homosexual urban areas.

Outreach work provides not only a perfect opportunity to promote services; it also provides a means of identifying and contacting some of those who are most vulnerable and at risk. Ben is one example; his story is similar to many of those using the Armistead's services.

Ben was first contacted in one of the bars on Liverpool's homosexual scene and was made aware of the services that the Armistead provided. A few weeks later, he presented to the service and slowly his story began to unfold. Ben had been emotionally, physically, and sexually abused as a child. His mother, a single parent, drank heavily and would lash out at him for no apparent reason. She entered into a relationship when Ben was six, and it was not long before her partner begun to sexually abuse him. When he finally disclosed the abuse, no one believed him.

> I didn't know what was happening, I was so young. I didn't know what was going on. My mum used to leave me with no food and I would be hungry. I spent most of my time locked in my bedroom. I never knew anything else. Soon the school started to come to find out why I wasn't in. I also got into trouble because they said I was talking about things sexual. No one picked up on it. One time my mother's boyfriend smashed my head against the wall, I was never checked out or anything. When I did tell about the abuse they all screamed at me and called me a liar. In the end it was easier to say I had dreamt it. At 13 I had had enough, I took myself off to Social Services and asked them to put me in care. I was then sent to a children's home in another city.

Ben remained in the children's home until he was 18, and was by this time using drugs such as ecstasy and cocaine recreationally. From an early age, he had already showed signs of having a mental health problem. He had self-harmed from the age of 10 and had suffered long periods of depression. When this culminated in a suicide attempt, the home professionals felt unable to cope with his behaviour and he was then asked to leave. Sent out to fend for himself, and with little support offered, he was ill-equipped to live on his own and his drug use escalated. He began to use amphetamine, ecstasy and cocaine on a daily basis, as well as consuming large amounts of alcohol. He spent most of his time partying and found he could offer sex for money to pay for his substance use.

> Getting into drugs helped me cope. It took all the painful memories away and I was just having a good time. I went wild and began sleeping around. I had no respect for myself, I was never sober when I had sex, I was always off me head.

Problematic substance use is something that affects a large proportion of people worldwide. Yet, we do not give much thought to the sexuality of those experiencing substance use problems, and how this impacts on their mental health and influences their substance use. In the two decades this author has spent working in the drugs field, I have never been aware of any data being collected regarding an individual's sexuality when being assessed for substance use treatment. Some may argue that it is unnecessary to know this information, while others may view this knowledge as important in supporting the individual on their life journey. Certainly, in Ben's case his sexuality played a major role in his lifestyle and the problems he was experiencing.

We know that substance use problems do not exist in isolation of other factors, and many experiences from childhood and adolescence may leave the individual vulnerable to some substances more than others. In Ben's case, his childhood experiences shaped his future, and attempting to block out his past, contributed to his chaotic lifestyle. A 2007, report[10] acknowledged that some individuals from the lesbian, homosexual, bisexual and transgender communities have a higher risk of mental disorder, suicidal behaviour and substance use. The report stated that despite a '*wealth of research evidence of increased risk of mental health and the greater use of services*', policy-makers appear to overlook the needs of these individuals.[10] Furthermore, they were not addressed in the UK National Suicide Prevention Strategy.[11] Such omissions begin to build a picture that, from governmental policy to service provision, there are huge inequalities.

It is hardly surprising then that individuals from the lesbian, homosexual, bisexual and transgender community are at higher risk of mental health and substance use problems. They are one of the most marginalised groups of people within most societies. It is estimated that 5% to 7% of the UK's population are lesbian, homosexual, bisexual and transgender,[12] yet there is little UK research regarding illicit substance use among these individuals. Some American and Australian studies, suggest that the individual from lesbian, homosexual, bisexual and transgender communities are twice as likely to have substance use problems than the general populations.[13] Despite this, successive mental health–substance use policy fails to mention, or even acknowledge, a sizeable group within the UK population. A report published by Sigma Research,[14] highlighted that homosexual men were being failed by substance use services, and those that did were 'poorly equipped' to help homosexual men.

If this is so, then clearly mental health–substance use services are falling short of addressing the needs of the individual from the lesbian, homosexual, bisexual and transgender communities. This may be, in part, due to an effect of entrenched homophobic views, moral standpoints and religious outrage and condemnation regarding acts of homosexuality. It appears that many professionals still fail to understand the culture and lifestyle of these individuals. While visiting one service, a professional from another suggested 'they' did not 'encourage' individuals to disclose their sexuality – '*If they're gay we tell them to keep it quiet*'.

> **KEY POINT 14.1**
>
> Stigma and shame attached to being lesbian, homosexual, bisexual and transgender is as prevalent today as it was prior to the decriminalisation of homosexuality in 1967 (UK).

This sends out a clear message that being homosexual is something that should remain hidden and secret – locked in 'the closet'. In some countries around the world today, being found guilty of acts of homosexuality can carry a death sentence and young lesbian, homosexual, bisexual and transgender people are being tortured on a daily basis simply because of their sexuality.

The 2008 Strategy 'Drugs: protecting families and communities'[15] acknowledges the gap in research regarding the service needs of those from homosexual communities. However, the strategy fails to address those needs, and in so doing, is not inclusive. The Sigma report[14] highlights that the majority of harms associated with substance use for homosexual and bisexual men, such as HIV transmission through unsafe sexual practices while under the influence of drugs, do not fit into the Home Offices definitions, nor are measurable using the Drug Harm Index.[16] The Index was developed to establish national indicators of harms associated with substance use by bringing together a range of measures of substance-related costs to individuals and society. One of the specified health harms relates to transmission of human immuno–deficiency virus (HIV) or hepatitis C virus (HCV) through injecting substances, heterosexual sex and neonatally. However, the strategy[15] has failed to recognise the role substance use plays in sexual HIV transmission among homosexual, lesbian and bisexual individuals, and is not included in the list of harms. It would appear that other indicators are as equally immeasurable. Therefore, demonstrating the need to extend or adapt the Drug Harm Index to encompass the needs of those from lesbian, homosexual, bisexual, and transgender communities that are vulnerable to substance harm from things other than opiates and intravenous substance use. The Sigma[14] team noted that the substance use strategy[10] was not orientated towards creating an infrastructure where the substance use among the lesbian, homosexual, bisexual, and transgender communities was addressed.

In Ben's case, his substance use not only affected his mental health, it impacted on his sexual health. He was diagnosed HIV positive at the age of 20. His substance use influenced his behaviour and, coupled with his low self-esteem and mental health problems, he did not practice – or even care – about his sexual health. By this time, he was back in his birth town and homeless, with very little support from any of the health and social care services when they were most needed. The service that had the most contact with him in this period of his life was Genito-urinary Medicine, and his experience there was far from satisfactory and appropriate to his needs.

> The health advisor from the clinic gave me my results over the phone. She had phoned me to tell me to come in to discuss my test results. I knew something was wrong, so I kept pushing for her to tell me what was

wrong. I was crying my eyes out when she said my HIV test had come back positive. But I was stopped in my tracks when she said to me, 'Well it's hardly a surprise given your lifestyle.' I just stopped crying. I thought these people were not supposed to judge you, I couldn't believe it. It just made me feel worse about myself. I didn't know what my future held or what was going to happen to me. I shouldn't have been told my results over the phone even though I pushed for it.

Ben felt judged by this professional, who may well have collected all the information on his sexual behaviour and substance use, but knew little of the circumstances that led him there. Gaining the individual's trust is paramount when working with the person experiencing mental health–substance use problems and the relationships formed play an important part in the helping process. It is vital that a non-judgmental approach is adopted. However, when dealing with individuals from the lesbian, homosexual, bisexual, and transgender communities being non-judgmental must also be applied to their sexual practices and preferences. Some professionals may find it uncomfortable talking about substance use, when drugs are specifically used to enable men to relax enough to engage in certain sexual acts, such as anal sex or 'fisting'. However, when working with lesbian, homosexual, bisexual and transgender communities it is important that one's own moral opinions and values do not creep in to working practices. Sadly, it is all too common to hear of anecdotal reports of inappropriate responses and judgemental attitudes. It also demonstrates that professionals have to be aware of how language and communication play a vital role in supporting the individual and addressing his/her needs.

What are the needs of this group? There are many things that can influence the mental health of individuals from the lesbian, homosexual, bisexual, and transgender communities. Given the levels of homophobia that exists in society, and the stigma attached to being homosexual, this a clear influence on self-esteem. With religious leaders condemning and castigating – and in some countries homosexual people are being denied even basic human rights, it is little wonder that this group is attracted to the escapism substance use offers. Certainly, substance use is an acceptable part of the social scene, despite the risks to physical, mental and sexual health.

One cannot discount the effect homophobia has on mental health. Many young homosexual people find themselves isolated from their families and friends who are unable to deal with the issues around sexuality. Often they will become homeless, as parents refuse to have anything more to do with their child for no other reason than them being 'gay'. Homelessness agency professionals in London estimated that 26% of young, street homeless identified as lesbian, homosexual, bisexual, and transgender.[17] They become victims of homophobic hate crimes and are often vulnerable to physical assault or murder. This author has found the sense of isolation homosexual people feel can at times be overwhelming. All the people this author has encountered during working practice have reported that they have been subjected to homophobic abuse at some time in their lives, if not on a daily basis. Substance use provides a quick fix for confidence, boost to self-esteem, and offers the means to escape from reality.

When the Armistead began working with Ben there were a number of issues to be addressed:

➤ housing
➤ substance use
➤ physical health
➤ mental health
➤ self-harm.

The trauma from childhood sexual abuse was still affecting Ben; by this time, he was also buying over-the-counter painkillers containing codeine and paracetamol (because he liked the 'floating feeling'). He took above the recommended dose, placing him at risk of liver damage. It was important that Ben was able to take an informed decision about the risks and appreciate the impact substance use was having on both his physical and mental health. It was also felt that referring him to a substance use service, may have made heroin more accessible.

> If I had gone to a drug service I would have ended up using smack [heroin] with all the others. I would have wanted to try it.

Together we looked at Ben's substance use, then discussed ways he could reduce the harm. It was explained that by using stimulant drugs regularly there was a possibility of his viral load increasing. Indeed this was later proved to be the case when on his next visit to the HIV clinic, following a cocaine binge, he was informed his viral load had increased from forty thousand to over half a million. He was made aware of how substances work on the brain and deplete certain brain chemicals, which enabled him to understand the negative impact this had had on his mental health. Harm reduction and substance interaction advice enabled Ben to make informed choices. Ben worked at his own pace, set his own goals, which later led him to stop using substances.

By attending medical appointments with him, Armistead advocated for Ben, and raised awareness of other health problems that concerned him, with appropriate health and social care professionals. Through the HIV clinic, he was able to access a psychologist to deal with the childhood trauma and move forward on these issues. While Ben has a long way to go, the positive experiences he has had from the Armistead professionals have gone a long way in helping him rebuild his life. Being able to talk to someone who understood not only his substance use, but also his lifestyle and sexuality made a huge difference. This may not have been possible in more generic mental health and substance use services. When working alongside lesbian, homosexual, bisexual and transgender individuals we have responsibility to ensure we are fully aware of the issues each individual faces, and to learn about each life, enabling effective delivery of services.

CONCLUSION

This chapter aimed to raise awareness of sexuality and sexual function. Hopefully, it has offered some guidelines on how to approach and develop services for this sensitive subject. The aim has been to help you:

1   recognise the importance of sexuality
2   listen to the individual's concerns
3   assess a situation and always review it
4   help to create a space for sexuality to be expressed and maintained
5   respect and support self-image
6   maintain the individual's dignity
7   use the expertise of the wider team.

One service development manager who has developed many strategies said:

> I have to ensure I include all the politically correct practices, words and phrases in mental health–substance use policy to meet the relevant regulations and targets. One day I would like to see such understanding and commitment working in practice!

The time for this is long past – but it is never too late to start to correct our professional skills, and offer inclusive interventions and treatment.

Harvey Milk,[18] an American campaigner for sexual equality said,

> If we are not free to be ourselves in that most human of all activities, the expression of love, then life itself loses its meaning!

ACKNOWLEDGEMENT

The first part of this chapter was adapted from Hibberd J. Sexuality in palliative care. © Cooper J. *Stepping into Palliative Care 1: relationships and responses.* 2nd ed. Oxford: Radcliffe Publishing; 2006. Reproduced with the permission of the copyright holder. The authors are grateful to Jo Cooper for permitting this adaptation.

DEDICATION

This chapter is dedicated to our friend and colleague, Phil Yates, who tragically took his own life and is now somewhere over the rainbow. Phil Yates, Area Project Worker, born 21 April 1980; died 18 May 2009.

REFERENCES

1   Cox K. Sexual identity – gender and sexual orientation. In: Oliviere D, Monroe B, editors. *Death, Dying and Social Differences.* Oxford: Oxford University Press; 2004.
2   Lawler J. *Behind the Screens.* Melbourne, VIC: Churchill Livingstone; 1991.
3   Rice AM. Sexuality in cancer and palliative care 1: effects on disease and treatment. *Int J Palliat Nurs.* 2000; **6**: 392–7.
4   Shell JA, Smith CK. Sexuality and the older person with cancer. *Oncol Nurs Forum.* 1994; **21**: 553–8.
5   Hughes MK. Sexuality and the cancer survivor. *Cancer Nurs.* 2000; **23**: 477–82
6   Antrobus S. Developing the nurse as a knowledge worker in health: learning the artistry of practice. *J Adv Nurs.* 1997; **25**: 829–35.
7   Dittemar S, editor. *Rehabilitation Nursing.* New York: Mosby; 1989.

8 Fogel CI, Lawer D. *Sexual Health Promotion*. Philadelphia, PA: WB Saunders; 1990.

9 The Armistead Centre. Available at: www.armisteadcentre.co.uk/ (accessed 9 June 2010).

10 Fish J. *Reducing Health Inequalities for Lesbian, Gay, Bisexual and Trans People: briefing for health and social care staff*. London: Department of Health; 2007. Available at: www.dh.gov.uk/en/Publicationsandstatistics/Publications/PublicationsPolicyAndGuidance/DH_078347 (accessed 9 June 2010).

11 Department of Health. *National Suicide Prevention Strategy for England*. London: Department of Health; 2002. Available at: www.dh.gov.uk/en/Publicationsandstatistics/Publications/PublicationsPolicyAndGuidance/DH_4009474 (accessed 9 June 2010).

12 Stonewall: the Lesbian, Gay and Bisexual Charity. *How Many Lesbian, Gay and Bisexual People are There?* 2008. Available at: www.stonewall.org.uk/at_home/sexual_orientation_faqs/2694.asp (accessed 9 June 2010).

13 Gilman SE, Cochran SD, Mays VM, *et al.* Risk of psychiatric disorders among individuals reporting same-sex sexual partners in the National Comorbidity Survey. *Am J Public Health.* 2001; **9**: 933–9.

14 Keogh P, Reid D, Bourne A, *et al. Wasted Opportunities: problematic alcohol and drug use among gay men and bisexual men*. London: Sigma Research; 2009. Available at: www.sigmaresearch.org.uk/files/report2009c.pdf (accessed 9 June 2010).

15 Home Office. *Drugs: protecting families and communities*. London: Home Office; 2008. Available at: www.emcdda.europa.eu/attachements.cfm/att_50809_EN_UK%20Strategy%202008-2018.pdf (accessed 9 June 2010).

16 MacDonald Z, Tinsley L, Collingwood J, *et al. Measuring the Harm from Illegal Drug Using – The Drug Harm Index*. Home Office online report 24/05; 2005. Available at: www.homeoffice.gov.uk/rds/pdfs05/rdsolr2405.pdf (accessed 9 June 2010).

17 Dunne G, Prendergast S, Telford D. Young, gay, homeless and invisible: a growing population? *Cult Health Sex.* 2002; **4**: 103–15.

18 Shilts R. *The Mayor of Castro Street: the life and times of Harvey Milk*. New York: St Martin's Press; 1982.

TO LEARN MORE

- Armistead Centre: www.armisteadcentre.co.uk/
- Centre for HIV and Sexual Health, Sheffield Primary Care NHS Trust, 22 Collegiate Crescent, Sheffield, S10 2BA UK. Operates nationally and locally. Tel: 0114 226 1900: www.sexualhealthsheffield.nhs.uk
- Nazarko I, Aylott J, Andrews A. Dilemmas: how should nurses respond to patients' sexual needs? *Nurs Times.* 2000; **96**: 35.
- Price B. A model for body image care. *J Adv Nurs.* 1990; **15**: 585–93.
- Roper N, Logan WW, Tierney AJ. *The Elements of Nursing*. 2nd ed. Edinburgh: Churchill Livingstone; 1990.
- Sigma Research: www.sigmaresearch.org.uk/go.php
- Webb C. Nurses' knowledge and attitudes about sexuality in health care. *Int J Nurs Stud.* 1987; **25**: 235–44.

CHAPTER 15

Mental health in the UK:
the legal dimension

Nicola Glover-Thomas

Comment:
Throughout this book (and book series) the term 'individual', 'person' and/or 'people', has been used instead of 'patient(s)', (unless a direct quote or reference to a text). However, for this chapter 'patient', remains for this enhances understanding and interpretation of this text. The reader is asked to be mindful that this term relates to an individual with concerns and dilemmas – just like us.

INTRODUCTION

This chapter will consider the role of law in mental healthcare provision under the Mental Health Act 1983,[1] as amended by the Mental Health Act 2007.[2] The main purpose of mental health legislation is to ensure that some patients suffering from a mental disorder (as defined) are forced to accept admission to hospital and/or compulsory treatment without their consent. The Mental Health Act 2007[2] sets out the criteria and procedures to be followed to enable that to take place. The Act permits both 'civil' hospital admissions as well as criminal justice admissions from the courts or prison. The primary focus in the 2007 Act[2] is on the presence of mental disorder and the risk posed by the patient to him/herself or others. The Act tries to strike a balance between individual autonomy and society's right to deprive that individual of their liberty. Most provisions of the 2007 Act came into force in November 2008. It represents the culmination of a protracted and controversial reform process, which began in 1998. The Mental Health Act 2007[2] was the Government's third attempt to introduce significant legislative changes to the Mental Health Act 1983,[1] following a decade of increasingly vociferous calls for the law to reflect more fully contemporary psychiatric practice.[a]

Since the 1950s, mental healthcare provision has moved progressively away from reliance upon institutionally focused care to a more flexible, community care-based model. Several policy drivers have motivated this less restrictive care approach, not least the expectation that costs to the state would be significantly reduced following such a care approach. In particular, inpatient facilities, including inpatient beds, have been shrinking year on year, with bed capacity in psychiatric units falling from 154 000 in 1954 to 32 400 in 2004.[4] Yet, despite such a clear evidential representation of the community care approach being fully endorsed, this reduction in hospital-based facilities has not been mirrored in compulsory admission figures of psychiatric patients under the legislation, which is (approximately) 250 000 per annum.[5] Compulsory admission under the Mental Health Act 1983 has steadily increased from less than 20 000 per year in the 1960s and 1970s, to over 27 000 per year in 2005–2006. These figures represent the still-growing phenomenon of the 'revolving-door patient', whereby large numbers of people with severe and often chronic mental illness are receiving primary care within the community yet are experiencing more frequent, though shorter, periods of inpatient care through the application of the Act. This legislation is increasingly required to act as a mechanism that offers mental health professionals the means to overcome acute episodes of mental distress experienced by patients in the community while mental health policy itself remains resolutely rooted within the community care ideology.

In addition to clear policy changes in psychiatric care that have been reflected in several amendment Acts since the Mental Health Act 1959,[b] awareness of the fundamentality of human rights and the need to protect these rights has become an inherent aspect to the legal process. The Human Rights Act 1998,[6] has played a significant role in the changing landscape of mental health law, bringing into sharp focus the necessity for public authorities to act compatibly with the European Convention on Human Rights. This raises particular difficulties in the mental health arena as mental health legislation necessarily provides legitimate means for mental health professionals to force patients to be admitted to hospital and to undergo treatment. Where it can be demonstrated that clinical decisions of this kind would be in the patient's own interests or for the protection of others, they are legally justifiable even when it is clearly against the patient's own will.

This balance between patient rights, the rights of others to protection and ensuring legal legitimacy remains paramount and strikes at the heart of the debate about mental health law reform. The Mental Health Act 2007[2] was the culmination of a lengthy and often uncertain process of reform that began in 1998 when the governments appointed an Expert Committee to review the 1983 Act. In the intervening nine years, several consultation papers, a White Paper in 2000 and the first draft bill in 2002 were published. Following a further lengthy and at times acrimonious period of consultation, a further draft Mental Health Bill was published in 2004. Both the 2002 and 2004 Bills were vigorously criticised and the 2004 Bill being substantially similar to the previous Bill was subject to sustained wholesale condemnation which was concluded by further criticism by the Joint Pre-parliamentary Scrutiny Committee. Following this, the Government decided to drop plans to repeal the Mental Health Act 1983,[1] and instead opted to introduce an amendment Act. The Mental Health Act 2007,[2] is effectively a statutory adjunct to the Mental Health Act 1983 and does not offer a comprehensive new code.

Despite continued efforts to establish an effective equilibrium between the protection of patient rights and the protection of the public, the 2007 Act has shifted clearly towards the enhancement of public protection mechanisms by emphasising risk management as a key objective. Among other things, powers, found in the 1983 Act, have been extended in relation to compulsion. The definition of mental disorder, the filtering device used to determine whether the mental health legislation should apply to individuals, has been significantly broadened. In addition, in an effort towards achieving a much more reflective legislative system that acknowledges the importance of the community as the primary care environment, compulsory community treatment orders have been introduced. The 2007 Act[2] emphasises that the focus of the legislation is that of ensuring people using the psychiatric care system comply with their care package including the acceptance of medication, even where the individual concerned is unwilling.

This chapter will review the changes brought about by the 2007 Act[2] and consider the wider implications that may flow from them. Consideration will be given to the 'new' definition of mental disorder, examining its wider scope. The implications of the new 'appropriate medical treatment' test will then be considered in conjunction with the detention criteria under the 2007 Act. The chapter will then go on to describe and analyse the new and wider roles and responsibilities of mental health professionals in the assessment, treatment and discharge process and an evaluation will be made of the new community treatment orders. Finally, a brief consideration will be given to the additional safeguards introduced by the 2007 Act.

THE GUIDING PRINCIPLES IN THE CODE OF PRACTICE

Section 118 of the 1983 Act,[1] places a duty on the Secretary of State (and the National Assembly in Wales) to prepare, and from time to time, revise a Code of Practice 'for the guidance' of those exercising functions in relation to the admission and treatment of patients under the 1983 Act. A revised Code was published in 2008 and there are five guiding principles outlined. They are intended to inform decisions made under the Act and provide guidance as to how the Act should be implemented. The guiding principles in the Code embrace the following:

1 **Purpose principle**: Decisions under the Act must be made with a view to minimising the undesirable effects of mental disorder, by maximising the safety and wellbeing of patients, promoting recovery and protecting other people from harm.
2 **Least restriction principle**: People taking action without a patient's consent must attempt to keep to a minimum the restrictions they impose on the patient's liberty.
3 **Respect principle**: People taking decisions under the Act must recognise and respect the diverse needs, values and circumstances of each patient, including their race, religion, culture, gender, age, sexual orientation and any disability.
4 **Participation principle**: Patients must be given the opportunity to be involved, as far as is practicable in the circumstances, in planning, developing and renewing their own treatment and care to help ensure that it is delivered in a way that is as appropriate and effective for them as possible.
5 **Effectiveness, efficiency and equity principle**: People taking decisions under the Act must seek to use the resources available to them and to patients in the most effective, efficient and equitable way, to meet the needs of patients and achieve the purpose for which the decision was taken.

Overall, paragraph 1.8 of the Code (para 1.8)[1] states that the principles are intended to inform decisions, but they do not determine them. The weight given to each principle in reaching a particular decision will depend on the context. Furthermore, in making decisions under the Act, the principles, as a whole, need to be balanced in different ways according to the particular circumstances of each individual decision.[7] That is not to say that any of the principles should be disregarded but, rather, the weight given to each one will depend upon the particular circumstances of the individual concerned.

The emphasis in the principles would seem to be on inclusivity, encouraging participation, respecting patients as individuals and promoting their dignity and autonomy wherever possible. Professionals are also reminded of the need to respect patient rights as the Code expressly advises that all decisions must be lawful which includes compliance with the Human Rights Act 1998.[6] Since the 1998 Act came into force, all public authorities are under a legal duty to make decisions which are compatible with the European Convention on Human Rights.

Fennell,[5] in paragraph 2.46, has noted that section 118 of the Act[6] now contains a list of 'matters' which must be taken into account by the Secretary of State in preparing the statement of principles in the Code. The list specifically includes the effectiveness of treatment and public safety. This will certainly include emphasis on compliance with medication and signals a shift towards seeking to ensure patient compliance with medication and risk management.[5] The first purpose principle also makes explicit reference to the need to make decisions under the Act which protect other people from harm. Arguably, therefore, the Code's commitment to patient rights and autonomy is not as strong as it appears. This is also evinced by the fact that the Richardson Committee had recommended that principles such as these should be included on the face of the Act itself, and the Parliamentary Joint Committee on Human Rights on the Draft Mental Health Bill[8] agreed. However, the government ultimately did not. This is regrettable, as the Mental Capacity Act (MCA) 2005,[9] stands in stark contrast to this. The emphasis in the MCA 2005 is undoubtedly on empowerment and personal autonomy which is made clear with the five principles on the face of the Mental Capacity Act itself. This suggests a dilution in the commitment towards empowerment and autonomy of mentally disordered patients in the Mental Health Act, and is much weaker than an explicit statutory requirement. This list is tucked neatly away in the Code of Practice and, as Fennell notes[5] 'is a good deal weaker than a statutory requirement to have regard to principles spelt out in statute, and crystallises the difference between the two statutes' (p. 37).[5] It remains to be seen how significant an effect they will have on the way the Act is operated and, in turn, what impact that will have on patient autonomy and treatment.

THE STATUS OF THE NEW CODE OF PRACTICE

Section 118(2D)[7] states that persons exercising functions under the Act should 'have regard' to the Code.[7] The relevance of the Code to decision-making was considered in the case of *(R) Munjaz v Mersey Care NHS Trust*.[10] The facts related to the use of seclusion in Ashworth Hospital and the applicant challenged its use in breach of the Mental Health Act Code of Practice. In this case, the majority of the House of

Lords found that the Code did not have the binding effect of a statutory provision or instrument. It is guidance and not instruction. Lord Bingham stated that:

> the Code does not have the binding effect which a statutory provision or a statutory instrument would have [but] . . . the guidance should be given great weight. It is not instruction, but it is much more than mere advice which an addressee is free to follow or not as it chooses. It is guidance which any hospital should consider with great care, and from which it should depart only if it has cogent reasons for doing so (para 21).[10]

Consequently, the Code should be observed by all professionals who are using the Act and hospitals cannot depart from it as a matter of policy. Cogent reasons could relate to a hospital departing from the Code in respect of groups rather than individual patients. This could be a policy decision arising from the special problems of high security hospitals, which contain the most potentially dangerous patients in the country. It could justify differences in the seclusion policy with respect to the special position of such patients whom it was necessary to seclude for longer than a very few days.

Section 118 should, therefore, be interpreted in accordance with this dictum. Accordingly, departures from the Code will be rare and there must be clear and convincing reasons for justifying such a departure.[c]

DEFINING 'MENTAL DISORDER'

Statutory definitions act as the initial filtering mechanism which effectively provides a remit for which the legislation will apply. In so doing, the population potentially affected and the scope of the legislation's applicability are demarcated. The definition of mental disorder under the Mental Health Act 1983,[1] was subject to sustained criticism largely because it offered a complicated and convoluted two-tier definition which affected the applicability of the admission provisions. Part I of the 1983 Act,[1] defined mental disorder by providing a general definition of mental disorder which was mental illness, psychopathic disorder, arrested or incomplete development of mind and *any other disorder or disability of mind*. This general definition was sufficient to allow for a section 2, admission for assessment, procedure which gave a 28 day power of admission for assessment only. The second tier of the definition provides specific categories:

➤ mental illness
➤ severe mental impairment
➤ mental impairment
➤ psychopathic disorder.

If an individual was thought to meet one of these specific definitions, then the 1983 Act granted the power to admit them to hospital for treatment for up to six months.

The 2007 Act,[2] abolishes the four separate definitional categories of mental disorder, which was required for longer-term admission under section 3. In its place, a single definition has been introduced which applies to all provisions within the

Act. The new, simplified definition of mental disorder is '*any disorder or disability of mind*'. Effectively, the 2007 Act[2] definition has followed on from the position adopted in the 1983 Act,[1] for the shorter stay admission for assessment provision (s 2) and acts as a 'bucket' category. This effort to broaden the definition and its applicational scope has largely been motivated to avoid previous problems with categories of individuals that have evaded the scope of the legislation in the past. Of particular concern to the Government was the perceived risk generated by individuals with personality disorders. The 1983 Act[1] definition required that the compulsory detention of such a group could only ever be legally justified if there was evidence of abnormally aggressive or seriously irresponsible conduct. Under the 2007 Act[2] all that is necessary is that '*appropriate medical treatment*', such as nursing and psychological therapy is available to them and that detention in hospital is necessary for their own health or safety or for the protection of others.

To ensure detention under the mental health legislation is compatible with Article 5(1) of the European Convention on Human Rights,[7] and hence, the Human Rights Act 1998,[6] certain conditions must be met. Article 5(1) provides that no one should be deprived of their liberty unless the deprivation is carried out in accordance with legal procedures. Article 5(1)(e) allows for the deprivation of liberty to be legally justified on the basis of unsoundness of mind. Such deprivation may be justified if the '*Winterwerp conditions*' are met.[11] It must be shown that the individual concerned can be reliably shown to be of unsound mind, based on objective evaluation; the mental disorder must be such to warrant compulsory confinement; and, that continued confinement can be justified on the basis of the mental disorder's persistency.

Detention based on the new definition of mental disorder under the 2007 Act,[2] must still meet the conditions laid down by *Winterwerp*.[12] However, the 2007 Act,[2] has removed the definitional exclusions that were present in the 1983 Act,[1] definition barring the 'drug and alcohol dependency' exclusion (s 1[3]). The sexual deviancy exclusion has been abolished, not in an effort to do a volte-face on the more liberal viewpoint adopted on sexual orientation, but rather to enable paraphilia within the definition should there be a need. In particular, paedophilia has become a greater concern for the Government in recent years and the sexual deviancy exclusion has, up until the 2007 Act,[2] effectively prevented any therapeutic responses to paedophilia being available within a compulsory environment.[e]

'APPROPRIATE MEDICAL TREATMENT' TEST

Under the Mental Health Act 1983,[1] the 'treatability test' played a crucial role in ensuring that the legislation remained purposive in character. In other words, given the need to protect potential rights, as being a fundamental aspect to the legislation, deprivation of liberty had to have a legitimate reason. The 'treatability test' applied to psychopathic disorder and mental impairment and in order for detention or renewal of detention, a doctor had to agree or certify that medical treatment was likely to alleviate or prevent deterioration in the patient's condition. In the decision of *Reid v. Secretary of State for Scotland*[13] 'treatment' was interpreted broadly and their Lordships were of the view that treatment could comprise any number of therapies and treatments. However, the Government remained sceptical that the 'treatability test' would never be used as a means of justifying a decision not to detain and this was particularly thought to be the case with individuals with personality disorders who refused to cooperate with treatment strategies. The concern in relation to patients with personality disorders was that it might be very difficult to prove a treatment has a valuable and overtly positive contribution to make to an individual's condition when the patient refuses to participate willingly.

Instead, the 2007 Act[2] merely requires that appropriate treatment must be available to an individual irrespective of whether it is willingly accepted or rejected. This change has been introduced in order to ensure that clinicians do not feel compelled to predict whether treatment would be effective in a given individual and in circumstances where such a prediction could not be made; the clinician decides not to detain. In addition, the change seeks to avoid the particular difficulties surrounding personality disorders where the individual may not be prepared to comply but who presents a risk to themselves or others nevertheless. A patient's refusal to accept treatment can no longer act as a barrier to detention as long as appropriate treatment is available.[f]

As noted by Fennell, the 'appropriate treatment test' applies regardless of whether the patient accepts the treatment.[5] Section 3(4) of the Mental Health Act as inserted by the 2007 Act[2] states that:

> References to appropriate medical treatment, in relation to a person suffering from mental disorder, are references to medical treatment which is appropriate in his case, taking into account the nature and degree of the mental disorder and all the other circumstances of his case.

According to the new Code of Practice,[g] 'all the other circumstances' includes factors, such as the patient's physical health and disability, the patient's age, culture, ethnicity, gender or sexual orientation as well as the location and implications of the available treatment (para 6.11).[7] The new broader definition of 'medical treatment' now includes 'psychological intervention and specialist mental health habilitation, rehabilitation and care' (s 7 of the 2007 Act).[2] This is not exhaustive so can include a broad range of treatments, including psychotherapy, drug therapy and electroconvulsive therapy (ECT).[h] It also means that patients with a personality disorder can receive appropriate behaviour and psychotherapy. The Code makes it clear that the definition includes treatment of physical health problems only to the extent that such treatment is part of, or ancillary to, treatment for mental disorder (para 23).[7] An example would be treating wounds self-inflicted as a result of mental disorder. All other medical treatment for physical health problems falls outside the Act and is regulated by the common law or the Mental Capacity Act 2005.[9]

The Law Society was concerned that 'specialist' intervention should include some level of supervision by a psychiatrist,[13] but this has not been clearly stated in the Act or Code of Practice. Consequently, it is not entirely clear whether this provision complies precisely with the European Convention on Human Rights requirement for objective medical expertise when a patient is receiving non-consensual medical treatment for a mental disorder. The Code expressly states that the purpose of this test is to ensure that no one is detained (or remains detained), or is a community patient unless they are actually to be offered medical treatment for their mental disorder (para 6.7).[7] The test requires a judgement about whether appropriate medical treatment is available given:

1 the nature and degree of the patient's mental disorder
2 all the other circumstances of the patient's case.[7] (para 6.10)

In other words, both the clinical appropriateness of the treatment and its appropriateness more generally must be considered.

This amendment has received a great deal of criticism from a number of campaign groups. For example, there is a concern that using availability of appropriate treatment as a basis for compulsory detention could be misused to exclude patients inappropriately from medical treatment due to the scarcity of mental health resources.[14] The fact that the Code states that '*it is not sufficient that appropriate treatment could theoretically be provided*' and that '*medical treatment must actually be available to the patient*' does seem to reinforce this point. There were also concerns that this test opened up the possibility for detaining people for whom there is no therapeutic benefit (para 3.1).[15] However, this fear is unlikely to materialise as the 2007 Act[2] has inserted a new subsection 4 into section 145 which makes it clear that 'medical treatment' must demonstrate some benefit in terms of being for the '*purpose of alleviat*[ing], *or prevent a worsening of, the disorder or one or more of the symptoms or manifestations*'. And paragraph 6.17 of the Code[7] makes it clear that simply detaining someone, even in a hospital, does not constitute medical treatment.

The Code of Practice stresses that purpose is not the same as likelihood, which means that there is no need to show in advance that the purpose is likely to be achieved (para 6.4).[7] Furthermore, and of particular relevance to the discussion about personality disorder, the Code reminds professionals that there may well be a range of interventions which are appropriate even if particular mental disorders are likely to persist or get worse despite treatment. In addition, '*it should never be assumed that any disorders, or any patients, are inherently or inevitably untreatable*' (para 6.6).[7]

PROFESSIONAL ROLES

The Mental Health Act 2007[2] has changed the professional roles and responsibilities of mental health decision makers. The Approved Mental Health Practitioner (AMHP), and the Responsible Clinician have effectively replaced the Approved Social Worker and the Responsible Medical Officer roles under the 1983 Act. The Approved Social Worker's role involved taking primary responsibility for making applications for compulsory admission to hospital and guardianship while the medical professionals' involvement under the Responsible Medical Officer role, took the form of providing medical recommendations for compulsory admissions, being responsible for compulsory in-patient treatment and making leave of absence and discharge decisions. Traditionally, the medical practitioners was always a consultant psychiatrist and usually held section 12[i] approval status which acknowledged them as having specialist experience in the diagnosis and treatment of mental disorder.

These roles have been overhauled under the 2007 Act[2] and perhaps most significantly the functions of both professional roles have now been opened up to a wider group of professionals, including nurses, occupational therapists and clinical psychologists, as well as social workers and psychiatrists. The motivation for this change is to allow different professionals who equally meet the skills and experience needed for such mental health decision-making to be able to participate fully in this role. This change is intended to *'remove the current demarcation of professional roles, in favour of a new approach which ensures that professionals with the right skills, experience and training can carry out important functions not currently open to them'* (para 3).[16] It has also been recognised as essential that modern mental health legislation is able to fully reflect contemporary healthcare practices and included within this is the need to recognise an increasingly 'integrated management approach' to decision-making. What the expansion of professional roles also does is to expand the professional pool that can be used to provide full responsibility for patients, once approval has been obtained.

The changes brought into being have not been accepted without some criticism. This criticism is focused particularly on the AMHP role, where there is significant concern that social workers who worked hard to establish and maintain an independent non-medical perspective[17] in the compulsion process could find this threatened with the opening up of the professional role. The other concern relates to the question of how much influence social workers are likely to be able to exert over other senior medical colleagues and the impact this could have on confinement decisions. There is a strong need for disciplinary and professional independence in order to ensure that the best interests of patients are met. Approved Social Workers have been independent from their own management but it has been reported that they *'frequently witness Health Service management interference in the clinical decision making of nurses, e.g. linking admission and discharge proposals to bed control targets'.*[18,19] Moreover, psychiatric nurses are in a *'formal hierarchical relationship with psychiatrists, bound to respond to their clinical instructions: in the view of Approved Social Workers, this would be incompatible with the civil liberties element of the role'.*[19] Peay, conducted extensive research into dual decision-making by mental health practitioners under the 1983 Act.[20] In total, 106 practitioners participated in the research, including consultant psychiatrists and Approved Social Workers. The research suggested that psychiatrists' individual preference for using compulsion was overwhelming (73%), whereas only 40% of the Approved Social Workers would have used compulsion in this way. This research suggests that Approved Social Workers can be effective and *'act as a brake on making decisions to invoke the Act'.*[20] Accordingly, diluting the involvement of Approved Social Workers in the compulsion decision could be detrimental to patients, possibly resulting in an increase in the use of compulsion at the expense of exploring other, less restrictive community based options.

COMPULSORY TREATMENT IN HOSPITAL

Part IV of the Mental Health Act 1983[1] was regarded as a revolutionary step towards the recognition and protection of patient rights. It introduced a legislative framework of powers which organised various treatments according to severity.

This framework allowed for the administration of treatment for mental disorder without the consent of the patient as long as the Second Opinion Appointed Doctor (SOAD) safety mechanism was in place. Section 57[1] provides that treatments of an irreversible nature, such as psychosurgery and surgical hormone implants, cannot be administered without both the patient's valid consent and a second medical opinion supporting the given treatment course. Unlike section 57, section 58 does authorise treatment without patient consent but is limited in its application to patient's who have been detained under powers which authorise detention beyond 72 hours. Patients who are detained under section 4 and are therefore viewed as emergency admissions and voluntary patients who are held under the section 5 'holding powers' are not covered by section 58. Furthermore, section 58 will not apply to patients who are conditionally discharged restricted patients and remand patients (under s 35).[1] Section 58, prior to the enactment of the Mental Health Act 2007,[2] covers medicines for mental disorder, and ECT. Such treatments can be administered under section 58 if either the patient consents to the treatment or a SOAD certifies that the patient is either unable to consent or is capable of consent but is refusing the treatment and that the proposed treatment should be administered anyway. When making this assessment, the SOAD was required to consider whether such treatment offered a means by which the patient's condition could be 'alleviated or deterioration prevented'. However, since the 2007 Act,[2] the 'treatability test' (as discussed above) has now been replaced by the 'appropriate medical treatment' test and as such, has widened significantly the parameters of the definition of medical treatment for mental disorder.

The Mental Health Act 2007[2] has also introduced one further change in relation to the powers to treat those with mental disorders. The 2007 Act has removed ECT from section 58 and its administration is now governed by a newly introduced section 58A. This provides that other than in emergencies where the administration of treatment is necessary to protect the patient's life or to prevent a serious and immediate deterioration in the patient's condition, ECT may not be given if the patient is mentally capable and is refusing to consent. Section 58A applies to patients who are detained under the powers which authorise detention beyond 72 hours and who are not conditionally discharged restricted patients or patients subject to remand under section 35. However, section 58A does apply to patients under the age of 18 who are voluntary and not subject to the legislation with proxy consent being sufficient.

Most significant about the changes brought about in relation to ECT is the introduction of an additional second medical opinion procedure. As noted above, section 57 requires the SOAD to certify the patient is able and willing to consent and that treatment is appropriate; whereas section 58 requires the SOAD to state that the patient is either incapable of consenting to the treatment or is capable and is refusing, but that treatment is necessary. While section 58A requires the SOAD to accept that where a patient is mentally capable but refusing treatment, ECT may not be given irrespective of his clinical views about the merit of the proposed treatment in the given case.

COMMUNITY CARE/TREATMENT: THE COMMUNITY TREATMENT ORDER

The introduction of the Community Treatment Order (CTO) must be seen as one of the most significant changes brought about by the 2007 Act.[2] The CTO was argued by the Government to offer the means by which the ever growing phenomenon of the 'revolving door patient', whereby patients improve in hospital, are discharged, stop taking their medication and relapse requiring re-admission, could be gradually eradicated. CTOs attempt to respond to this peripatetic behaviour by providing closer supervision in the community. It is also intended to reduce the risk of social exclusion, which is associated with detention in hospital for long periods of time (page 3).[16] A patient can now be placed on a CTO after one period of inpatient detention and effectively, the patient will live within the community though will remain under the control of the legislation and mental health decision makers. Considerable practical concerns remain about how realistic the CTO will prove to be and just how successful and easy to use the treatment provisions in conjunction with the CTO will be.

Part 4A of the Mental Health Act 1983[1] regulates the administration of 'relevant treatment' of community patients whilst they remain in the community. Section 62A governs the treatment process for patients who are recalled back to hospital whilst on a CTO. Essentially, the CTO works on the basis that any treatment given to patients while they are subject to a CTO requires patient consent and a certification by a SOAD authorising the treatment. Where a patient refuses treatment under a CTO, treatment may only be given without consent by recalling the patient back to hospital and treating them under section 62A.

If a community patient is recalled under section 17E, or where the CTO is revoked under section 17F, section 62A applies. The patient is treated as if he remained liable to be detained since the CTO was first created. However, for treatment to be justifiable under section 58, a certificate given by a SOAD must exist or must be arranged quickly. For patients recalled to hospital because of refusal of treatment within the community, for the purposes of section 58 the patient must already be the subject of a certificate covering section 58 treatment that was made prior to the CTO being arranged. If a certificate exists, there will be no necessity to acquire a new one. Likewise, if the period from when the patient first received medication during detention and the period under the CTO is less than three months, the original certificate will suffice. However, what is necessary is that the certificate must make clear that the treatment specified is appropriate on recall following a CTO. Changes in clinically assessed need regularly feature within care and treatment planning and this must be acknowledged and accounted for, if necessary. Where treatment has not been specified, then treatment cannot be given on recall unless the proposed treatment's administration is covered by Part 4.

It is also worth noting that for patients for whom ECT is considered the most appropriate treatment strategy, a Part 4A certificate will not provide the necessary legal authority to justify section 58A treatment when the patient has capacity to consent but refuses to do so.

Where a patient remains in the community under a CTO, section 64A–64K govern the circumstances when treatment for mental disorder may be given in the community. Clearly, if the patient has capacity to consent and is willing to take their medication in the community, few legal or practical difficulties are likely to emerge. However, some scope has been incorporated into the Mental Health Act 2007[2] to allow treatment to be administered in the community to patents who do not provide the necessary consent because they are incapable of doing so. Circumstances that may allow for treatment in the community without consent are:

➤ if consent is given by someone authorised under the Mental Capacity Act 2005[9] to make decision on the patient's behalf

➤ when the patient lacks capacity but no force is required to ensure compliance with the administration of the medication; or

➤ where emergency treatment is needed, using force if necessary, to an incapable patient.

Where the above conditions cannot be met, any treatment against the will of a community patient will be unlawful.

NEW SAFEGUARDS

A brief examination must be given to the other changes to the Mental Health Act 1983[1] which seek to offer the patient additional safeguards when subject to the legislation. The 2007 Act[2] has made a number of changes to the role of the nearest relative, who has the power to apply for compulsory admission and challenge the patient's compulsory detention. The nearest relative is determined by virtue of a statutory list which has been modified by the 2007 Act to include civil partners as well as same or opposite sex couples living together as man and wife. As result of a successful challenge to the 1983 Act under the Human Rights Act 1998,[6,j] the 2007 Act has also introduced a new provision to enable the patient to seek displacement of an unsuitable nearest relative.

A key development in the 2007 Act[2] has been the introduction of Mental Health Advocates to provide support for certain groups of detained patients, guardianship patients and patients subject to supervised community treatment,[k] with the exception of those held under sections 4, 5, 135 or 136. Section 30(2) places a duty on the Secretary of State (or Welsh Assembly) to provide advocacy services, which includes help in obtaining information about and understanding the provisions of the Act and why they have been applied. Advocacy also includes help in obtaining information about any rights which may be exercised in relation to the patient. Advocacy is perceived to be an important protection for the patient. There is also a duty on service providers to provide qualifying patients with information that advocacy services are available – for patients on guardianship this is likely to be channelled through the Approved Mental Health Practitioner and it will be the responsibility of the hospital managers for patients liable to be detained.[21 table 34.2] Under section 130(D) of the 1983 Act, Approved Mental Health Practitioner will have a duty to take whatever steps are practicable to ensure patients understand that help is available to them from independent mental health advocates (IMHAs) and how they can obtain that help. This must include giving the relevant information both orally and in writing.[21 para 34.20] Independent mental health advocates will have a duty to visit and interview a patient if requested to do so by an AMHP, the patient's nearest relative or responsible clinician (s 130B[5]).[1] Independent mental health advocates will also have the right to interview professionals and look at records, provided it is for the purpose of supporting the patient (s130B[3] and [4])[1]. Although advocacy services have been available for a while, they have not been monitored and there are national variations in quality and quantity. Consequently, the new advocacy provisions will be introduced gradually from April 2009 to allow time for guidance, training, and capacity to develop.

Another important mechanism for safeguarding patients and standards of mental healthcare is perceived to be the Mental Health Act Commission. It was established in the 1983 Act[1] as a multidisciplinary and independent body to monitor and oversee the use of compulsory powers in the Act. The Commission has carried out regular hospital inspection visits, investigates the handling of complaints made by detained patients and produces biennial reports. Significantly, the Mental Health Act Commission has now been abolished and its functions transferred to the Care Quality Commission, a new integrated health and social care regulator. This step, which came into force in April 2009, brings together existing health and social care regulators into one body.

A final important patient safeguard is the Mental Health Review Tribunal. Tribunals were introduced by the Mental Health Act 1959 to provide patients with an opportunity to seek independent review of their continued detention. The tribunal system was left largely untouched by the 2007 Act and the only changes relate to the system of automatic reviews where a patient has not applied for review and the establishment of separate Tribunals for England and Wales. However, the passing of the Tribunals, Courts, and Enforcement Act 2007 has led to the recent replacement in England of the Mental Health Review Tribunal by a new First Tier Tribunal.

CONCLUSION

The 2007 Act[2] amends the 1983 Act[1] and sets out a new framework for determining when and how people will be subject to the use of compulsory powers. It has made a number of significant changes. These changes seek to offset some of the perennial difficulties with the Mental Health Act 1983, which have hampered good mental healthcare delivery in the past. To what extent these changes will be successful remains to be seen, yet what is clear is that despite the introduction of several safeguards to protect the rights and needs of patients the primary focus of the legislation has shifted markedly towards risk assessment and management. The focus of reform since the 1990s was placed on risk as a key factor in the compulsion decision, introducing more effective compulsory community powers and ensuring that dangerous and severely personality disordered patients could be subject to detention in the mental health system. As noted by Fennell, '[since] *the 1990s successive governments have pursued a public safety agenda in relation to mental health services responding to concerns about homicides by mentally disordered people*' (para 6).[7] The 2007 Act[2] is the culmination of this ongoing journey towards the harnessing of risk assessment processes. To what extent this legislative shift will influence mental health decision makers in their assessment of patients and how they respond to patients is subject to current ongoing research[1] but it can only be hoped that experienced professional judgement will not be overshadowed too greatly by the public safety agenda.

REFERENCES

1 Department of Health. *Mental Health Act 1983*. Available at: www.dh.gov.uk/en/ Publicationsandstatistics/Legislation/Actsandbills/DH_4002034 (accessed 9 June 2010).

2 Department of Health. *Mental Health Act 2007*. Available at: www.dh.gov.uk/en/Healthcare/ Mentalhealth/DH_078743 (accessed 9 June 2010).

3 Bartlett P, Sandland R. *Mental Health Law: policy and practice*. Oxford: Open University Press; 2007.

4 Warner L. *Beyond the Water Towers: the unfinished revolution in mental health services 1985–2005*. London: Sainsbury Centre for Mental Health; 2005.

5 Fennell P. *Mental Health: The new law*. Bristol: Jordans; 2007.

6 Human Rights Act 1998. Available at: www.direct.gov.uk/en/Governmentcitizensandrights/ Yourrightsandresponsibilities/DG_4002951 (accessed 9 June 2010).

7 Department of Health. *Revised Code of Practice 2008 Department of Health Code of Practice: Mental Health Act 1983*. Revised ed. London: The Stationery Office; 2008. Available at: www. dh.gov.uk/prod_consum_dh/groups/dh_digitalassets/@dh/@en/documents/digitalasset/ dh_087073.pdf (accessed 9 June 2010).

8 Joint Committee of Human Rights. Session 2001–02 Joint Committee of Human Rights: Twenty-fifth Report. Available at: www.publications.parliament.uk/pa/jt200102/jtselect/ jtrights/181/18104.htm (accessed 9 June 2010).

9 Department of Health. *Mental Capacity Act 2005*. Available at: www.dh.gov.uk/en/SocialCare/ Deliveringadultsocialcare/MentalCapacity/MentalCapacityAct2005/DH_073511 (accessed 9 June 2010).

10 *Munjaz v Mersey Care NHS Trust* [2003] 3 WLR 793.

11 *Winterwerp v Netherlands* (application 6301/73) (1979) 2 EHRR 38–7.

12 *Reid v Secretary of State for Scotland* (1999) 1 All ER 482.

13 Bell A. T*he new mental health law still does not do justice to the patients*. Parliamentary Brief; 23 July 2007. Available at: www.parliamentarybrief.com/2007/07/the-new-mental-health-law-still-does-not-do-justice (accessed 9 June 2010).

14 Law Society. *Mental Health Bill Second Reading, House of Lords, Tuesday 28 November 2006*. Available at: www.mentalhealthalliance.org.uk/policy/documents/LawSociety_Bill_ Lords_2R_Briefing.pdf (accessed 9 June 2010).

15 Royal College of Psychiatrists Briefing on the Mental Health Bill. *Welfare Reform Bill 2009 Royal College of Psychiatrists Second Reading Briefing House of Commons*. Available at: www. rcpsych.ac.uk/pdf/RCPsych%20Welfare%20Reform%202nd%20Reading%20briefing%20 Jan09.pdf (accessed 9 June 2010).

16 Department of Health. *Mental Health Bill 2006: summary guide*. London: Department of Health; 2006. Available at: www.dh.gov.uk/en/Publicationsandstatistics/Publications/ PublicationsLegislation/DH_062926 (accessed 9 June 2010).

17 Fawcett B. Consistencies and inconsistencies: mental health, compulsory treatment and community capacity building in England, Wales and Australia. *Br J Soc Work*. 2007; **37**: 1027–42.

18 Walton P. Reforming the Mental Health Act 1983: an approved social worker perspective. *J Soc Welf Fam Law*. 2000; **22**: 401–14.

19 Brown R. The changing role of the approved social worker. *J Ment Health Law*. 2002; December: 392–8.

20 Peay J. *Decisions and Dilemmas Working with Mental Health Law*. Oxford: Hart; 2003. pp. 16, 47.

21 Department of Health. *Reference Guide to the Mental Health Act 1983*. London: The

Stationery Office; 2008. Available at: www.dh.gov.uk/en/Publicationsandstatistics/
Publications/PublicationsPolicyAndGuidance/DH_088162 (accessed 13 April 2010).

NOTES

a   Owing to a lack of space, this chapter will focus on the civil procedures within the mental
health legislation alone; mentally disordered offenders are given admirable treatment elsewhere in Bartlett P and Sandland R. *Mental Health Law: policy and practice.* Oxford: Oxford
University Press; 2007.

b   These are: the Mental Health (Amendment) Act 1982 which consolidated with the Mental
Health Act 1959 and brought about the Mental Health Act 1983; the Mental Health (Patients
in the Community) Act 1995; the Human Rights Act 1998; the Mental Capacity Act 2005;
and the Mental Health Act 2007.

c   For further discussion *see* Bowen P. *Blackstone's Guide to the Mental Health Act 2007.* Oxford
University Press; 2007. pp. 58–60.

d   The removal of the exclusions, including that of sexual deviancy, from the definition of
mental disorder under the 2007 Act seeks to counter such situations arising in the first
place, see *Reid* [1999] 1 All ER 482.

e   In *R (on the application of MN) v. Mental Health Review tribunal* [2007] EWHC 1524. The
patient argued that the MHRT should discharge him on the basis that the only component
of his psychopathic disorder that he engaged in was his paedophilic tendencies and as these
were acts in pursuit of his sexual deviancy it would fall within the 1983 Act's exclusions.
This argument was rejected and upheld.

f   Section 145 of the 2007 Act outlines what medical treatment amounts to – it includes
nursing and psychological care, as well as specialist mental habilitation, rehabilitation and
care.

g   The Mental Health Act 1983, revised Code of Practice (Department of Health Code of
Practice Mental Health Act 1983 (2008). The revised Code had a commencement date of
3 November 2008.

h   Special rules and procedures apply to certain treatments, such as ECT, medication beyond
an initial three-month period, neurosurgery and surgical hormone implants (ss 57, 58,
58A).

i   A section 12 doctor is one who is approved as having special knowledge and experience in
the diagnosis and treatment of mental disorder. The formal detention processes under the
Mental Health Act 1983 required two medical recommendations for compulsory admission
to the hospital under sections 2 and 3, of which one recommendation must have been made
by a section 12 approved doctor. This stringent evidential standard in the formal detention
process remains under the Mental Health Act 2007.

j   *See JT v United Kingdom* (2000) 30 EHRR CD 77, ECtHR.

k   *See* further, ss 130A–D Mental Health Act 1983.

l   Research is currently being conducted by the author into initial institutional and individual
responses to the Mental Health Act 2007, in relation to the perceived risk profiles of patients
and responding decision-making of service providers.

Useful chapters

The Mental Health–Substance Use series comprises six books. To develop knowledge and understanding chapters are interlinked, building and exploring specific areas. It is hoped the following will help readers locate relevant chapters easily.

BOOK 1: INTRODUCTION TO MENTAL HEALTH–SUBSTANCE USE
1 Setting the scene
2 Learning to learn
3 What is in a name? The search for appropriate and consistent terminology
4 The mental health–substance use journey
5 A matter of human rights: people's right to healthcare for mental health–substance use
6 The importance of physical health assessment
7 The experience of illness
8 The psychological impact of serious illness
9 Working with people with mental health–substance use
10 Skills, capabilities and professional development: a response framework for mental health–substance use
11 Attitudes and brief training interventions: a practical approach
12 Ethics: mental health–substance use
13 Brain injury, mental health–substance use
14 Heatwave, mental health–substance use

BOOK 3: RESPONDING IN MENTAL HEALTH–SUBSTANCE USE
1 Setting the scene
2 The family perspective
3 The individual's perspective: hard to reach people or hard to access services?
4 The female perspective
5 The older adult's perspective
6 The young person's perspective
7 The child's perspective
8 The additive effect of mental health–substance use on cognitive impairment

Useful contacts

Collated by Jo Cooper

Addiction Arena – www.addictionarena.com
Addiction Medicine – http://listserv.icors.org/SCRIPTS/WA-ICORS.
    EXE?A0=ADD_MED
Addiction Rehabilitation Facilities – www.arf.org/isd/bib/mental.html
Addiction Technology Transfer Center – www.nattc.org/index.html
Addiction Today – www.addictiontoday.org
Alcohol and Alcohol Problems Science Database – http://etoh.niaaa.nih.gov
Alcohol and Drug History Society – http://historyofalcoholanddrugs.typepad.com
Alcohol Concern – www.alcoholconcern.org.uk/servlets/home
Alcohol Drugs and Development – www.add-resources.org
Alcohol Focus Scotland – www.alcohol-focus-scotland.org.uk
Alcohol Misuse (Department of Health) – www.dh.gov.uk/en/Publichealth/
    Healthimprovement/Alcoholmisuse/index.htm
Alcohol Reports – www.alcoholreports.blogspot.com
Alcohol, Other Drugs and Health: Current Evidence – www.bu.edu/aodhealth/index.
    html
Alcoholics Anonymous – www.aa.org
Alcoholism and Substance Abuse Providers – www.asapnys.org
American Psychiatric Association – www.psych.org
American Society of Addiction Medicine – www.asam.org/CMEonline.html
ATTC Network – www.attcnetwork.org/index.asp
Australasian Professional Society on Alcohol and other Drugs – www.apsad.org.au
Australian Drug Foundation – www.adf.org.au
Australian Drug Information Network – www.adin.com.au/content.asp?Document_ID=1
Australian Government Department of Health and Ageing:
Alcohol – www.alcohol.gov.au
Illicit drugs – www.health.gov.au/internet/main/publishing.nsf/Content/healthpubhlth-
    strateg-drugs-illicit-index.htm
Mental health – www.health.gov.au/internet/main/Publishing.nsf/Content/mental-pubs-
    npol08
Australian Professional Society on Alcohol and Other Drugs – www.apsad2008.com
Berman Institute of Bioethics – www.bioethicsinstitute.org
Best Practice Portal – www.emcdda.europa.eu/best-practice

BioMed Central – www.biomedcentral.com

Brain Injury Australia – www.bia.net.au

Brain Trauma Foundation – www.braintrauma.org

Brief Addiction Science Information Source – www.basisonline.org/2007/10/toward-a-balanc.html

Campaign for Effective Prevention and Treatment of Addiction – www.solutionstodrugs.com/index.htm

CEBMH – www.cebmh.com

Centre for Addiction and Mental Health – www.camh.net

Centre for Addiction and Mental Health: Mental Health and Addiction 101 Series – www.camh.net/MHA101

Centre for Clinical and Academic Workforce Innovation – Tel: 01623 819140. Email: ccawi@lincoln.ac.uk

Centre for HIV and Sexual Health, Sheffield Primary Care NHS Trust – www.sexualhealthsheffield.nhs.uk

Centre for Independent Thought – www.centerforindependentthought.org

Centre for Mental Health – www.scmh.org.uk/index.aspx

Clan Unity – www.clan-unity.co.uk

Committee on Publication Ethics – http://publicationethics.org

Communities of Practice for Local Government – www.communities.idea.gov.uk

Community Nursing Network – www.communitynursingnetwork.org/

Comorbid Mental Health and Substance Misuse in Scotland – www.scotland.gov.uk/Resource /Doc/127665/0030583.pdf

Creative Commons – http://creativecommons.org

Daily Dose: drug and alcohol news from around the world – http://dailydose.net

Dartmouth Psychiatric Research Centre – http://dms.dartmouth.edu/prc/dual

Department of Health – www.dh.gov.uk

Department of Health. *Mental Health Policy Implementation Guide: dual diagnosis good practice guide*. London: Department of Health; 2002 – www.dh.gov.uk/en/Publicationsandstatistics/Publications/PublicationsPolicyAndGuidance/DH_4009058

Department of Primary Health Care – www.primarycare.ox.ac.uk/research/dipex

Doctors.net.uk – www.doctors.net.uk

Drink and Drugs News – www.drinkanddrugs.net

Drinks Media Wire – www.drinksmediawire.com/afficher_cdp.asp?id=2625&lng=2

Drug and Alcohol Findings – http://findings.org.uk

Drug and Alcohol Nurses of Australia – www.danaonline.org

Drug and Alcohol Services, South Australia – www.dassa.sa.gov.au

Drug Misuse Information Scotland – www.drugmisuse.isdscotland.org/smrt/smrt.htm

DrugInfo Clearinghouse – http://druginfo.adf.org.au

Drugs and Mental Health –www.thesite.org/drinkanddrugs/drugsafety/drugsandyourbody/drugsandmentalhealth

Drugtext Internet Library – www.drugtext.org

Dual Diagnosis – www.hoseahouse.org/infirmary/dualdx.html

Dual Diagnosis Support Victoria – http://dualdiagnosis.ning.com

Dual Diagnosis Toolkit – www.rethink.org/dualdiagnosis/toolkit.html

Dual Diagnosis Website – http://users.erols.com/ksciacca
Dual Diagnosis: Australia and New Zealand – www.dualdiagnosis.org.au/home
Enter Mental Health: www.entermentalhealth.net/home2.html
European Alcohol Policy Alliance – www.eurocare.org
European Association for the Treatment of Addiction – www.eata.org.uk
European Federation of Nurses Associations – www.efnweb.org/version1/en/index.html
European Monitoring Centre for Drugs and Drug Addiction – www.emcdda.europa.eu
European Working Group on Drugs Oriented Research – www.dass.stir.ac.uk/old-site/
    sections/scot-ad/ewodor.htm
Eye Movement Desensitisation and Reprocessing Training Workshops – www.
    emdrworkshops.com
Faces and Voices of Recovery – www.facesandvoicesofrecovery.org
Federation of Drug and Alcohol Professionals – www.fdap.org.uk/certification/dap.html
Global Alcohol Harm Reduction Network – http://groups.google.com/group/
    gahrnet?hl=en&pli=1
Global Health Council – www.globalhealth.org
Guardian UK: the most useful websites on dual diagnosis – http://society.guardian.co.uk/
    mentalhealth/page/0,8149,688817,00.html
Headway – www.headway.org.uk
Health and Safety Executive (HSE) – www.hse.gov.uk/stress
HIT – www.hit.org.uk
Horatio: European Psychiatric Nurses – www.horatio-web.eu
Hub of Commissioned Alcohol Projects and Policies – www.hubcapp.org.uk
Inexcess: in search of recovery – www.inexcess.tv
International Brain Injury Association – www.internationalbrain.org
International Centre for Alcohol Policies – www.icap.org
International Council of Nurses – www.icn.ch
International Council on Alcohol and Addictions – www.icaa.ch
International Drug Policy Consortium – www.idpc.net
International Harm Reduction Association – www.ihra.net
International Nurses Society on Addictions – www.intnsa.org
International Society of Addiction Journal Editors – www.parint.org/isajewebsite/index.
    htm
IVO: scientific institute in lifestyle, addiction and related social developments –
    www.ivo.nl
James Lind Library – www.jameslindlibrary.org
Join Together: advancing effective alcohol and drug policy, prevention and treatment –
    www.jointogether.org
Madness and Literature Network – www.madnessandliterature.org/index.php
Medical Council on Alcohol – www.m-c-a.org.uk
Medline Plus – www.nlm.nih.gov/medlineplus/dualdiagnosis.html
Mental Health (About.com) – http://mentalhealth.about.com
Mental Health and Addictions Research Network – www.mhanet.ca/index.php
Mental Health Europe – www.mhe-sme.org/en.html
Mental Health Forum – www.mentalhealthforum.net/forum
Mental Health Foundation – www.mentalhealth.org.uk/welcome

Mental Health in Higher Education – www.mhhe.heacademy.ac.uk/sitepages/educators/?edid=239

Mental Health Information for All (RCPSYCH) – www.rcpsych.ac.uk/mentalhealthinfoforall.aspx

Mental Health Research Network – http://homepages.ed.ac.uk/mhrn

Middlesex University Dual Diagnosis Courses – www.mdx.ac.uk/courses/postgraduate/nursing_midwifery_health/index/aspx

MIND: for better mental health – www.mind.org.uk

Ministry of Justice: National Offender Management Service – www.justice.gov.uk/about/noms.htm

Mood Disorders Association of Canada – www.mooddisorderscanada.ca

Motivational Interventions for Drugs and Alcohol Misuse in Schizophrenia – www.midastrial.ac.uk

Motivational Interviewing – www.motivationalinterview.org

National Alliance on Mental Illness (US) – www.nami.org

National Centre for Education and Training on Addiction Australia – www.nceta.flinders.edu.au/index.html

National Comorbidity Initiative Australia – www.health.gov.au/internet/main/publishing.nsf/Content/health-pubhlth-publicat-document-metadata-comorbidity.htm

National Consortium of Consultant Nurses in Dual Diagnosis and Substance Use – www.dualdiagnosis.co.uk

National Drug and Alcohol Research Centre – http://ndarc.med.unsw.edu.au

National Drug Research Institute – http://ndri.curtin.edu.au

National Health Service – www.nhs.gov.uk

National Health Service Litigation Authority – www.nhsla.com/home.htm

National Institute for Health and Clinical Excellence – www.nice.org.uk

National Institute of Mental Health – www.nimh.nih.gov

National Institute on Alcohol Abuse and Alcoholism – www.niaaa.nih.gov

National Institute on Drug Abuse – www.drugabuse.gov/nidahome.html

National Treatment Agency for Substance Misuse – www.nta.nhs.uk

New Directions in the Study of Alcohol – www.newdirections.org.uk

New South Wales Health Dual Disorders resources – www.druginfo.nsw.gov.au/illicit_drugs

NHS Institute for Innovation and Improvement – www.institute.nhs.uk

Nordic Council for Alcohol and Drug Research (NAD) – www.norden.org/en/areas-of-co-operation/alcohol-and-drugs

O'Grady CP, Skinner WJ. A Family Guide to Concurrent Disorders. Toronto: Centre for Addiction and Mental Health; 2007. – www.camh.net/Publications/Resources_for_Professionals/Partnering_with_families/partnering_families_famguide.pdf

Partnership in Coping – www.pinc-recovery.com

PROGRESS: National Consortium of Consultant Nurses in Dual Diagnosis and Substance Use – www.dualdiagnosis.co.uk

Promoting Adult Learning – www.niace.org.uk/current-work/area/mental-health

Psychiatric Nursing – www.citypsych.com/index.html

Psychminded – www.psychminded.co.uk

Public Access (National Institutes of Health) – http://publicaccess.nih.gov/index.htm

Rethink (UK) – www.rethink.org/dualdiagnosis
Royal College of General Practitioners – www.rcgp.org.uk
Royal College of Psychiatrists – www.rcpsych.ac.uk
Royal Society for the Encouragement of Arts – www.thersa.org/home
SANE Australia – www.sane.org
Schizophrenia Society of Canada – www.schizophrenia.ca
Scholarship Society – www.scholarshipsociety.org
Scottish Addiction Studies – www.dass.stir.ac.uk/sections/showsection.php?id=4
Scottish Addiction Studies Library – www.drugslibrary.stir.ac.uk
Social Care Institute for Excellence – www.scie.org.uk
Social Care Online – www.scie-socialcareonline.org.uk
Society for the Study of Addiction – www.addiction-ssa.org
Spanish Peaks Mental Health Centre – www.spmhc.org
Stigma in Mental Health and Addiction – www.cmhanl.ca/pdf/Stigma.pdf
Substance Abuse and Mental Health Center toolkit for integrated treatment
     for co-occurring disorders – http://mentalhealth.samhsa.gov/cmhs/
     CommunitySupport/toolkits/cooccurring
Substance Abuse and Mental Health Data Archive – www.icpsr.umich.edu/SAMHDA
Substance Abuse and Mental Health Services Administration – www.samhsa.gov
Substance Misuse Management in General Practice – www.smmgp.org.uk
The Addiction Project – www.theaddictionproject.com
The Clifford Beers Foundation. Promotion of Mental Health –
     www.cliffordbeersfoundation.co.uk/jcont91.htm
The Co-occurring Centre for Excellence (US) – www.coce.samhsa.gov
The International Community for Hearing Voices – www.intervoiceonline.org
The International Network of Nurses – www.tinnurses.org
The International Society for the Study of Drug Policy – www.issdp.org
The James Lind Alliance Guidebook – www.jlaguidebook.org
The Management Standards Consultancy – www.themsc.org
The Mentor Foundation – www.mentorfoundation.org/about_mentor.
     php?nav=3-27-34-150
The Methadone Alliance Forum – www.m-alliance.org.uk/forum.html
The National Centre on Addiction and Substance Abuse – www.casacolumbia.org/
     templates/Home.aspx?articleid=287&zoneid=32
The National Treatment Agency – www.nta.nhs.uk
The Oxford Centre for Neuroethics – www.neuroethics.ox.ac.uk
The Recovery Workshop – www.recoveryworkshop.com
The Royal College of Psychiatrists. Changing Minds Campaign – www.rcpsych.ac.uk/
     campaigns/previouscampaigns/changingminds.aspx
The Sacred Space Foundation – www.sacredspace.org.uk
The United Nations Office on Drugs and Crime – www.unodc.org
The University of Toronto Joint Centre for Bioethics Centre for Addiction and Mental
     Health Bioethics Service – www.jointcentreforbioethics.ca/partners/camh.shtml
Tidal Model – www.tidal-model.com
Tilburg University, Department of Tranzo – www.uvt.nl/tranzo
Toc H – www.toch-uk.org.uk

Treatment Improvement Exchange – www.treatment.org

Trimbos Institute: Netherlands Institute on Mental Health and Addiction – www.trimbos. org

Turning Point – www.turning-point.co.uk

Tx Director – www.txdirector.com

UK Database of Uncertainties about the Effects of Treatment – www.library.nhs.uk/ DUETs/Default.aspx

UK Drug Policy Commission – www.ukdpc.org.uk/index.shtml

UNGASS – www.ungassondrugs.org

US Department of Health and Human Services. Co-occurring Mental and Substance Abuse Disorders: a guide for mental health planning + advisory councils. Alexandria, VA: National Association of Mental Health Planning and Advisory Councils; 2001 – http://download.ncadi.samhsa.gov/ken/pdf/NMH03-0146/ NMH03-0146.pdf

Victorian Alcohol and Drug Association – www.vaada.org.au

Web of Addictions: links to other websites related to addiction – www.well.com/user/ woa/aodsites.htm

Wired In: empowering people – http://wiredin.org.uk

World Health Organization (Management of Substance Abuse) – www.who.int/substance abuse/en

World Health Organization (Mental Health Policy) – www.who.int/mental_health/ policy/en

World Health Organization: Global Change and Health – www.who.int/globalchange/en/

World Medical Association – www.wma.net/en/10home/index.html

Youth Drug Support, Australia – www.yds.org.au

Index